D0254702

Th Gluten Syndrome

Is wheat causing you harm?

Dr Rodney Ford
MD MBBS FRACP

Are you being damaged by gluten?

At last your illness has been recognized and
now there is a name for it: *The Gluten Syndrome*.

Gluten is found in foods made from wheat, rye and barley.

Gluten can seriously affect your health by harming
your gut, your skin, and your nerves.

One-in-ten people are affected by gluten.
Are you the one?

The Gluten Syndrome
Is wheat causing you harm?

Copyright 2008 RRS Global Ltd.
Author: Dr Rodney Ford

National Library of New Zealand Cataloguing-in-Publication Data
Ford, Rodney, 1949-
The gluten syndrome : is wheat causing you harm? /
Rodney Ford ; illustrations by Liz Fazakarley.
Includes bibliographical references.
ISBN 978-0-473-12472-4
1. Gluten—Health aspects. 2. Celiac disease. 3. Food allergy.
I. Fazakarley, Liz, 1976- II. Title.
616.975—dc 22

Published by RRS Global Ltd.
PO Box 25-360, Christchurch, New Zealand.
www.doctorgluten.com
Printed by Tien Wah Press, Singapore
Second Printing, 2008
First printed 2007

All rights reserved.
Without limiting the rights under the copyright reserved above,
no part of this publication may be reproduced, stored in or
introduced into a retrieval system, or transmitted, in any form or by
any means (electronic, mechanical, photocopying, recording
or otherwise), without the prior written permission of the copyright
owner and the publisher of this book.

Jacket cover, art work and illustrations
by Liz Fazakarley of *Ford Design*.

Dedication

To my family, friends and patients who,
with open minds, have encouraged me and
who have made this work a possibility.

To you, the reader in the hope that,
with an open mind, you might feel the vibrancy
and health that your life has to offer.

"Where observation is concerned,
chance favours only the prepared mind."

Louis Pasteur, 1854

Other books with Dr Rodney Ford

The energy effect: your questions answered

Are you gluten-sensitive? Your questions answered

The book for the sick, tired and grumpy

Full of it! The shocking truth about gluten

Going gluten-free: how to get started

The gluten-free lunch book

Gluten-free parties and picnics

Eczema! Cure it!

Contents

Foreword

At last, all of the pieces of the gluten puzzle have been put together. The completed picture is "The Gluten Syndrome". It has taken over fifty years for the whole picture to be seen.

Many gluten suffers will rejoice that they now have their own syndrome. They will feel relieved that their condition now has an official medical label.

But others will be infuriated. A storm of controversy will rage. The defenders of coeliac disease will not like their disease being consigned to "The Gluten Syndrome".

The Gluten Syndrome has many supporters. Dr. Ron Hoggan has commented about the nerve and brain theory of gluten, when he reviewed Dr. Rodney Ford's book "Full of It! The shocking Truth about Gluten'. He wrote:

"A compelling new idea has dawned on the medical/scientific horizon. Dr. Rodney Ford, a pediatric gastroenterologist in New Zealand, who calls himself "doctorgluten" on the Internet, has come up with a startling hypothesis that synthesizes and makes sense out of a wide range of otherwise confounding findings in the celiac and gluten sensitivity literature. For instance, why have Dr. Marios Hadjivassiliou and his group found that some people with neurological disease with anti-gliadin antibodies but without celiac disease, recover on a gluten-free diet?"

"And why do other neurology patients sometimes recover from their neurological problems after treatment of their coexisting celiac disease? (Sadly, as Dr. Ford points out, by the time neurological disease develops the prognosis is often very poor.) Further, why do so many celiac patients present with such a wide range of symptoms, most of which are not obviously or usually associated with gut disease? And why are so many individuals who suffer from psychiatric, autoimmune, and even some infectious diseases, helped by a gluten-free diet?"

"The answer to all these questions, according to Dr. Ford's hypothesis, is that the primary gluten-driven disease is primarily an affliction of the brain. Gluten proteins and/or derivative peptides reach the brain and cause neurological damage along with hormonal and neurotransmitter abnormalities. The nerves in the gut, about as voluminous as the brain, are also damaged by these proteins and peptides."

"The net result is a cacophony of signs, symptoms, and manifestations across a broad range of organs and body systems. From epilepsy to abdominal distress to schizophrenia, gluten induced damage to the brain and connected nerve fibers can and does disrupt virtually any and every part of the body."

Ron Hogan concludes, "Dr. Ford credits a number of research heroes of gluten-related medical research, including Dr. Curtis Dohan, Dr. Marios Hadjivassiliou, Dr. Michael N. Marsh, Dr. Alessio Fasano, Dr. W.T. Cooke, Dr. A De Sanctis, Dr. Kenneth Fine, Dr. G.K.T. Holmes, Dr. A-M Knivsberg, Dr. Kalle Reichelt, and a host of others too numerous to list."

"Without doubt, Dr. Ford has 'seen further because he was standing on the shoulders of these giants,' (to paraphrase Sir Isacc Newton's famous statement). Nonetheless, Dr. Ford's novel view of this mass of research findings has led to his well supported hypothesis - one that threatens to overturn the current conception of gluten mediated disease."

"The symmetry and beauty of Ford's insight comes, in part, from its simplicity. It explains why there are so many and such varied manifestations of gluten sensitivity while making a minimal number of assumptions. And that, according to the long-standing principle of science called Occam's Razor, is the best possible explanation for a particular phenomenon."

It was in 1950 that Prof W. K. Dicke published his thesis "Coeliac disease: investigation of the harmful effects of certain types of cereal on patients suffering from coeliac disease". In this he asks, "If one acknowledges the existence of the wheat element (gluten), then one can investigate systematically the sensitivity of various groups with regard to wheat."

"In the clinic, one finds many sub-acute forms of enteritis and dyspepsia which respond poorly to normal therapy but well to wheat deprivation. Do these fall into the same category as the forme frustes of coeliac disease?"

Dicke's enquiry into the wide range of symptoms, which he had observed from gluten-sensitivity, were not answered. This was because the focus has been on the small bowel biopsy over the last 40 years. However, the argument has now turned full circle. The publication of "The Gluten Syndrome" has at last recognised the work of Dicke, and also incorporates both coeliac disease and more common reactions to gluten

Prof Ron Harper, Professor of Neurobiology, has this to say on the subject of gluten and the symptoms that it can casue, "This newly discovered link between gluten and the brain explains a number of recent phenomena associated with the syndrome. Both ADHD and autism have increased over the last few decades, paralleling the increase in the fast food industry which mass-produces foods that are loaded with gluten. Gluten may be a major contributor to these rising numbers of neurological difficulties."

"Epidemiology studies show that more than ten percent of the population show elevated IgG antibodies to gluten. This means that more than one in ten people are sensitised to gluten. Many of these people are likely to suffer from some degree of brain dysfunction caused by their reaction to gluten. The particular body symptoms expressed depends on the site of injury to the brain induced by gluten."

"The very high incidence of neurological disorders that are related to blood vessel regulation issues, including headaches, or directly related to cerebellar issues, such as attention deficit aspects, or disorders of movement or gait suggest that injury processes should be an object of attention. Any inflammatory process, such as found in response to sensitivity to gluten, should be suspect."

"It seems to me that gluten is a strong candidate for causing widespread neurological damage."

Ron Hoggan
Ed.D. Author, teacher and a diagnosed celiac who lives in Canada.
Author of the book "Dangerous Grains".
www.DangerousGrains.com

Ronald M. Harper
Ph.D. Distinguished Professor of Neurobiology,
David Geffen School of Medicine at UCLA,
University of California at Los Angeles.

Willem Dicke
PhD. Was Professor, Director of the Wilhelmina Children's Hospital,
Utrecht
Netherlands.

"There is nothing permanent except change."

Heraclitus

About the author

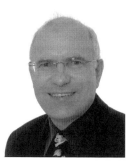

Dr Rodney Ford
Professor
MB BS MD FRACP MCCCH ASM

Dr Rodney Ford is a paediatric gastroenterologist, allergist and nutrition consultant. He is a former Associate Professor of Paediatrics at the Christchurch School of Medicine, University of Otago, New Zealand, and is recognized worldwide as an expert on adverse food reactions.

His major area of interest is the relationship between your food and your health – good or bad. In his clinics he is constantly seeing people who are suffering from eating foods that are making them ill. Gluten-sensitivity (or gluten intolerance) has long been a focal point of his investigations.

He believes that new knowledge should stimulate new thinking, and wants you to understand the new thinking about gluten-sensitivity and its multiplicity of symptoms. As a result of his research, Dr Ford believes that much of the damage caused by gluten is due to impairment of the brain and nerve networks. He calls this *The Gluten Syndrome.*

Dr Ford graduated with Honours from the University of New South Wales in 1974 (MB BS). He went on to study food allergy and intolerance problems in New Zealand, Australia and the United Kingdom, was admitted as a Fellow of the Royal Australasian College of Physicians in Paediatrics (FRACP) in

1981 and was awarded his Doctorate of Medicine (MD) by the University of New South Wales in 1982 for his thesis *Food hypersensitivity in children: diagnostic approaches to milk and egg hypersensitivity*. This was regarded as a major work on the diagnosis of food allergies in children.

Dr Ford currently runs the *Children's Gastroenterology and Allergy Clinic*, a busy private clinic in Christchurch, New Zealand. He has written over one hundred scientific papers, including book chapters and entire books. This book is the seventh in a series of books on the effects of gluten and what to do about it.

The seven books in the series are:
o   Are you gluten-sensitive? Your questions answered
o   Going gluten-free: how to get started
o   The gluten-free lunch book
o   Gluten-free parties and picnics
o   The book for the sick, tired and grumpy
o   Full of it! The shocking truth about gluten
o   The gluten syndrome: is wheat causing you harm?

The Gluten Syndrome

The Gluten Syndrome refers to the cluster of symptoms that you experience if you react to gluten. About one in ten people – tens of millions worldwide – are affected by *The Gluten Syndrome* – but few are aware of their plight. It's hard to know whether it is the gluten in the food you are eating that is making you sick unless you have the necessary knowledge. The purpose of this book is to tell you all about gluten, the harm that gluten can cause, and most importantly, what you can do about it.

This book presents you with the medical data and evidence behind the theory that gluten reactions are common – and serious. The story behind *The Gluten Syndrome* is disturbing. My prediction is that once there is worldwide recognition of the horrors of gluten, there will be a revolution in medical practice, in the field of mental health, and in food technology.

Tens of millions affected

Petrea King, founder of the *Quest for Life Centre*, wrote this about one of my seminars on gluten: "I'm sure that there will be a far-felt impact from your presentation as many of the practitioners have expanded their understanding of gluten sensitivities. In a hundred years your peers will consider what you know as 'common sense'. In the meantime, we admire your tenacity and commitment to pursue the cutting edge of real science."

To understand *The Gluten Syndrome* you need to know what gluten is and where it can be found; how gluten can make you sick; what symptoms you can attribute to gluten; how you can make a diagnosis; and what steps you need to take so that you can avoid gluten in your everyday life.

Rapidly accumulating evidence shows that gluten is now creating a massive health problem throughout the Western world, however woefully few people are aware of the catalogue of harm that gluten is causing.

The gluten link goes unrecognized

It is entirely possible that gluten could be responsible for one-third of all cases of chronic illness and fatigue. People suffering from these conditions are currently just putting up with their symptoms, unaware that gluten is the culprit. This is because the link to gluten has not yet been recognized by the medical community.

Gluten-containing products are being added to our food chain in ever-increasing amounts, and our wheat, which is one of the primary sources of gluten, is being genetically engineered to provide an even higher gluten content. This gluten overload is occurring while our communities remain unaware of the harm that this is causing.

Gluten can cause malfunctions of the brain and neural networks of susceptible people. The incidence of mental, neurological and brain disorders is on the rise, however the diagnosis of gluten-sensitivity is seldom made.

Gluten can damage brains

Gluten and other food intolerances are very common, and yet the medical system rejects the notion that common foods can be making you sick. Research shows that gluten causes significant symptoms in one in every ten people, but sadly, these people don't know that their symptoms can be cured simply by changing their diet.

Yes, the idea of *The Gluten Syndrome* is controversial. The concept is yet to be accepted by most 'mainstream' medical practitioners, however the evidence presented in this book provides overwhelming proof that gluten is causing countless numbers of people enormous misery and harm.

The community is already embracing the notion of gluten-sensitivity, and more and more people are opting for a gluten-free lifestyle. These people are looking for a term to identify their illness. Their search is over. They have been affected by *The Gluten Syndrome*. The time has come to lay out the evidence.

Do you have *The Gluten Syndrome?*

1. The pieces of the puzzle

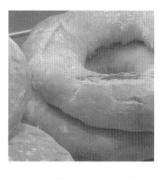

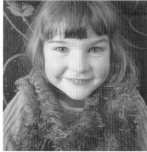

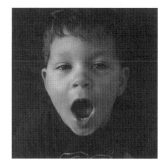

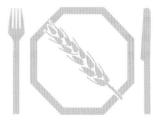

1. The pieces of the puzzle

"Real knowledge is to know the extent of one's ignorance."

Confucius.

Life can sometimes be seen as a giant puzzle that you spend your whole life solving. There seem to be thousands of pieces, and it can often take a while to figure something out as you struggle to make sense of it all.

Can you remember being told something by your parents, only to find out later that they had been wrong? You discovered that they had told you that your puzzle piece went 'there', but you found out some time later that it fitted somewhere else. Life is further complicated by the fact that while we are assembling our puzzle, we don't know how big the picture will be, what it will eventually look like, or even how many pieces we have to put together.

Medical puzzles

The study of medicine is a constantly evolving puzzle. New discoveries are being made all the time, which is like making even more pieces to fit into the puzzle. To make it more difficult, the picture that you are trying to put together is also changing. With each new insight into how the body works, new understandings emerge about how your body can get sick – and how your body can be healed. But the medical fraternity does not like to change the picture. Most organisations, including the medical hierarchy, strive to maintain the status quo – any change is strongly resisted.

Consequently, it takes a crisis or an accumulation of pent-up frustration to trigger a radical change. In the case of gluten, I dared to challenge the status quo in August 1990. I began to doubt the medical picture that I had been taught. The existing doctrine concerning gluten was that a gluten-free diet could only be instigated in someone who had been diagnosed with coeliac disease. A new way of looking at the gluten puzzle came into my life in the form of a little girl called Elizabeth.

Look at the gluten puzzle

At that time I was a consultant paediatrician doing gastroenterology and food allergy clinics in the Department of Paediatrics, Christchurch, New Zealand. I had been fully indoctrinated into the prevailing thinking regarding coeliac disease during a four-year training stint in the Department of Gastroenterology at the Royal Children's Hospital in Melbourne.

Elizabeth's gluten story

The first clue about *The Gluten Syndrome* – the link between gluten and poor health, independent of coeliac disease – appeared when I met Elizabeth. Her mother brought Elizabeth to my gastroenterology clinic on 23rd January, 1989. Elizabeth was a tiny six-year-old, short and thin for her age, with a big, bloated tummy. She had recently started at a new school, and was miserable. She was always complaining about her sore tummy, and burped and refluxed (sicked up) constantly.

Can gluten cause more than coeliac?

Previously, she had been thoroughly investigated by a number of paediatricians who had been looking specifically for coeliac disease, however they were unable to make that diagnosis because all her bowel tests, including tests for malabsorption and two small bowel biopsies, had been normal. Various medications had been tried, but they were not making any difference. Her doctors could offer no explanation, and Elizabeth's mother was becoming increasingly desperate.

Mother felt desperate

As I listened to her mother telling me this distressing story, I wondered if Elizabeth could have a gluten reaction in her oesophagus (gullet). Hers was an odd story, because she had all of the symptoms of coeliac disease, and yet her tests (including the two small bowel biopsies) were normal. I pondered what was happening – and wondered if gluten could be the cause of her reflux and pain.

With this novel possibility in mind, I suggested that Elizabeth try a gluten-free diet for a few months to test my theory. The family had reached crisis point and felt they had nothing to lose, so they agreed to cut out gluten from Elizabeth's diet.

Suggesting that someone who had not been proven to have coeliac disease should go on a gluten-free diet was seen as a heretical action. The decision was not condoned by my senior colleagues, who felt that it was not the thing to do in a teaching hospital – I could be leading the students astray!

However I had been working in the area of food allergy for the previous ten years, therefore I felt comfortable prescribing exclusion diets, both for children and entire families.

Elizabeth better in days!

To our amazement, within days Elizabeth was feeling immensely better! Both she and her mother were overjoyed. In my medical notes, I wrote: 'A new girl. Looks different. School teachers and ballet teacher can see the difference. No more swallowing of food all the time. More vital. When she strayed a little from her diet and ate gluten, she burped again for 24 hours.'

A remarkable recovery

Elizabeth was kept gluten-free and made a remarkable recovery. She began to grow again, she made new friends, and she was able to stop all her medications. In short, she was completely cured by adopting a gluten-free diet! One of my file notes reads: 'Sticking to her gluten-free diet. As soon as she has a deviation, she gets reflux. Had a few wheat-based cupcakes one day, and had reflux the next day. Took a week to fully recover. Otherwise, completely gluten-free.'

Gluten makes her ill

Elizabeth continued to remain gluten-free as she progressed through childhood and adolescence. She is now in her mid-twenties and continues to enjoy good health, although she still gets tummy pains and regurgitates food if she accidentally eats gluten.

Mum tells the story

Not long ago, her mother, Susan, sent me this note:

"As you can see, this recent photo of Elizabeth shines with the health and vitality which she has been blessed with over the past 15 years. This was not always so.

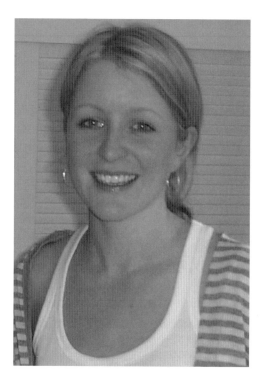

Soon after she was born, Elizabeth developed a reflux problem. She was a delightful baby during the day, but was plagued by colic at night. She suffered a 'near-miss' cot death at four months of age and was admitted to hospital for testing. It was concluded that she had choked as a result of having refluxed, as a similar incident occurred while she was in the ward.

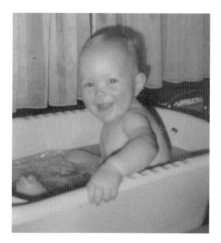

Despite this, Elizabeth continued to thrive until I stopped breastfeeding her when she was two years old. To our horror, her reflux became much worse, resulting in poor weight gain and stunted growth. She appeared to be very malnourished and her eyes were sunken, with enormous dark circles underneath them.

She became lethargic, prone to fainting at breakfast time, and vomited constantly at night, although she never complained. We put it down to her sweet nature, but perhaps she just didn't have the energy.

Elizabeth saw two paediatricians frequently over the following few years. Various tests were performed and a range of medicines were prescribed, with little or no effect. By now she was coughing up small amounts of dried blood, and we were feeling desperate. Surgery was contemplated to correct a supposedly faulty stomach valve.

When Elizabeth was six years old, we were transferred to Christchurch, and were fortunate enough to be referred to Dr Rodney Ford. It proved to be a wonderful meeting. I was enormously relieved by his interest in food intolerances, as I had raised this issue with the previous paediatricians, to no avail.

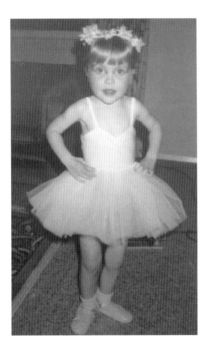

Dr Ford told us there was a new blood test available that could detect reactions to gluten. After conducting another bowel biopsy to check for signs of coeliac disease, Dr Ford told us that while Elizabeth had not suffered any gut damage from gluten, she did have an abnormal gluten blood test. For the first time, gluten was under suspicion as the cause of Elizabeth's problems.

We began Elizabeth on the gluten-free diet immediately, and the results were staggering. After just three weeks gluten-free, she was no longer vomiting during the night. A few weeks later, her reflux had completely disappeared. Her skin glowed, her eyes sparkled, and she became bubbly and energetic, excelling at ballet and sports. Over the next six months, she grew nearly 8cm in height.

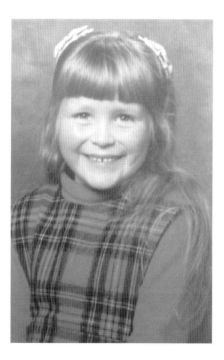

She was a new girl, and we were ecstatic! Teachers, friends and our family were stunned by her transformation. The most amazing thing was, the solution was so simple – no medication or surgery required!

Elizabeth is now 24 years of age, 170cm (5'7") tall, and working as a primary school teacher with special-needs children in London. She tries to stay gluten-free at all times, and knows when she has cheated (or been misled) because she develops a rash across her forehead.

We are forever grateful for Dr Ford's commitment to our daughter and his resolve to find an answer to her problems. We can't thank him enough, and wish him well with his research."

New pieces of the gluten puzzle

All those years ago, there was only one blood test available to help in making this diagnosis. This was the gluten antibody test (IgG-gliadin antibody test). The experience with Elizabeth began to change my approach to gluten. I had seen a child who did not have coeliac disease, but who had made a complete recovery by following a gluten-free diet.

This experience opened my mind, and I began to ask why gluten could make someone so unwell. I also began to seriously question the dogma of coeliac disease. There were new pieces to be added to the gluten puzzle, and the picture was definitely changing. It was then that I began the quest that has led to the discovery of *The Gluten Syndrome*.

Elizabeth has *The Gluten Syndrome*

2. Who dares disturb the giant?

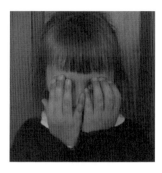

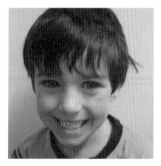

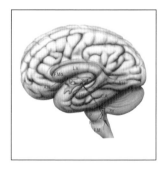

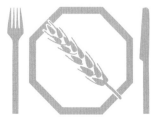

2. Who dares disturb the giant?

A hundred years of coeliac disease

The diagnosis and investigation of coeliac disease has a long tradition, having been the subject of intense investment by the medical profession for more than a hundred years. In that time, it has become the classic diagnosis in gastroenterology. As a result of this long history of medical research, it is now very difficult for the medical fraternity to acknowledge, let alone accept, a new angle on gluten. To fully understand the huge vested interest of the profession in protecting this iconic disease, first one must understand the 'sequence effect'.

The sequence effect

Each of us lives from day to day, and from hour to hour. Our lives have a sequence. The sun rises, and then the sun sets. We are used to experiencing our world as an orderly sequence of events.

Think about the photos and pictures that are hanging in your house, or your office. You probably thought carefully about where to hang them, and placed these pictures quite deliberately. You then hammered in a picture hook, because once hung, a picture is seldom moved. Recently, I was staying with friends and was amused to see the fading prints on their walls – they must have been there for several decades. They also had a few newer pictures for which wall space had somehow been found, but the old prints had not been moved. It seems that once the decision has been made to hang a picture, it becomes a life sentence! This is a perfect example of the sequence effect. As paintings and prints are accumulated over time, they are hung sequentially, and there they stay, never to be moved again. Not until a move of house, or a complete redecoration, occurs do these artworks come down from the walls and undergo a long-overdue repositioning. It takes a revolution to affect a change.

The same is true for the evidential picture for coeliac disease. As the medical evidence has been accumulated over the last century, each new piece has been carefully and deliberately hung on the walls of the existing ivory tower. Although much of this evidence is now faded and out of date, it continues to be clung to out of a sense of tradition. There has been a lot of emotional energy expended in hanging up, and hanging on to, these millions of pieces of data.

Gluten has been captured by coeliac researchers

Careers have been built investigating coeliac disease, and a gigantic structure of evidence has been built to define and explain the disease. The accepted dogma in most medical circles is that gluten causes coeliac disease, and nothing else. Gluten is located exclusively within the domain of coeliac disease, and it is not allowed to cause any other sickness. Who would dare to disturb this slumbering giant?

What is coeliac disease?

Coeliac disease is all about a tissue diagnosis. To make a diagnosis of coeliac disease, the gastroenterologist passes an endoscope tube through the mouth, through the stomach, and into the upper part of the small intestine. A small piece of tissue is snipped off and studied under a microscope. If the tissue is seen to be damaged, then you have coeliac disease. And if the tissue looks normal, then there can be no diagnosis of coeliac disease.

This reliance on a tissue diagnosis is a legacy from days gone by, before gluten blood tests were available. Fifty years ago, when blood tests were not yet available, the only way to obtain a diagnosis was to obtain a sample of the abnormal tissue. I believe that this has held back our understanding of how gluten causes harm. The focus on coeliac disease involved making a diagnosis that was solely based on tissue sampling (biopsy). The clinical symptoms have become irrelevant in making the diagnosis! In fact, many coeliacs have no symptoms at all.

One hundred years of coeliac disease

The history of coeliac disease extends over more than a hundred years, indeed descriptions of patients with diarrhoea and bloated abdomens have been found dating back over two thousand years.

The changes in the diagnostic approaches to coeliac disease are outlined in Diagram on the next page. The columns depict the three different approaches to the diagnosis of coeliac disease: clinical observation; small bowel biopsy; and blood tests. Unfortunately, each of these approaches has provided different, and often conflicting, information, hence the difficulties!

32

Changes in the diagnostic approach to coeliac disease over the history of one hundred years

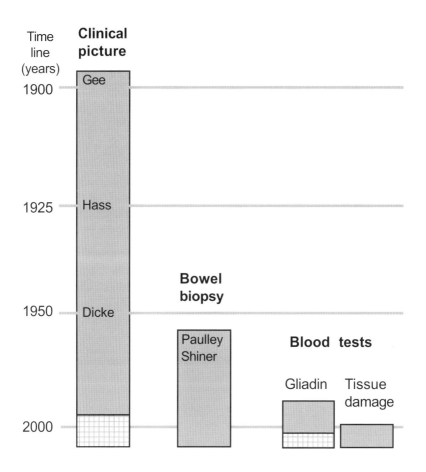

Legend:
The three diagnostic indicators are depicted by the columns:
Clinical picture; Bowel biopsy and Blood tests.
Grey shading depicts primary diagnostic indicators over time.
Light shading depicts less reliance now placed on the indicator.

The clinical picture

Dr Samuel Gee is acknowledged as the first person to name and comprehensively describe the clinical features of coeliac disease. In a lecture he presented in 1888 at the Hospital for Sick Children in Great Ormond Street, London, he accurately described the features of the illness. He also spoke of a digestive disorder, and wondered if this condition was related to food: "If the patient can be cured at all, it must be by means of diet." He described children between 1-5 years of age who were pale, and had thin, emaciated limbs and swollen bellies. They also produced loose, bulky stools and had a short life expectancy.

It must be emphasised that this was solely a clinical description – the cause was unknown, and the pathology was yet to be discovered. There were no blood tests or bowel tests available to assist with diagnosis in those days.

Subsequent refinements to Gee's clinical description were made by a number of people. In 1924, Haas recognised that grains might be to blame, and introduced his famous banana diet, which was used for many years until the introduction of the gluten-free diet.

Gluten was found to cause lots of symptoms

It was Dutch paediatrician Dr Willem Dicke who discovered that gluten was the central piece of the coeliac puzzle. Dicke published his findings in 1950 in his MD thesis *Coeliac disease: investigation of the harmful effects of certain types of cereal on patients suffering from coeliac disease.* He demonstrated that, in cases of children with coeliac disease, symptoms disappeared with the removal of wheat from their diet.

Dicke attributed this discovery, the link between coeliac disease and wheat flour, to the observations of the mothers of these sick children, however he was an astute observer himself. He began to see more and more illnesses that he suspected might be attributed to gluten.

In his thesis, he concludes: "In the clinic, one finds many sub-acute forms of enteritis and dyspepsia which respond poorly to normal therapy but well to wheat deprivation ... one could combine these cases under the term pre-coeliac disease." The spectrum of gluten-related reactions was starting to broaden.

The small bowel biopsy findings

The small bowel biopsy was the next landmark. It was John Paulley, a physician from Ipswich, who in 1954 first described the damaged appearance of the small bowel in patients with coeliac disease. These small bowel tissue biopsies were taken during abdominal operations. Paulley showed the typical loss of normal villi, which are finger-like projections on the bowel surface. This condition is now called villous atrophy (a full description of these changes can be found in my book *Are you gluten-sensitive? Your questions answered*).

With this discovery, the pace of investigation quickened and two years later, in 1956, Dr Margot Shiner developed a method whereby gut tissue samples could safely be obtained via the oral route. These biopsies involved taking a tiny piece of tissue from the lining of the upper bowel, the jejunum. The following year, the 'Crosby Capsule' was conceived and developed by an officer in the United States Army. This technique was used to perform these biopsies for the next thirty years until the fibre-optic endoscope was invented and its use became widespread. Nowadays, all small bowel biopsies are obtained by endoscopy.

Biopsy saga

As you can appreciate from the foregoing discussion, gastroenterologists have focused on the discovery of tissue damage for the last 50 years or thereabouts. Indeed, in order for a formal and definite diagnosis of coeliac disease to occur, an abnormal biopsy continues to be mandated – it is considered a *sine qua non*. In fact, the biopsy's appearance has overridden the importance of the patients' symptoms, which have become almost irrelevant to the gluten discussion.

Biopsy results suppressed the value of symptoms

This is a complete turnaround from the initial period when clinical descriptions were paramount. It now goes like this: if you have all of the symptoms of coeliac disease, but happen to have a normal biopsy, then you do not have coeliac disease. On the other hand, if you have no symptoms whatsoever, but return an abnormal biopsy, then you definitely have coeliac disease. To my mind, this sounds ridiculous; such an interpretation has lost sight of the larger gluten puzzle.

Biopsy thinking is flawed

This focus on the small bowel biopsy has three serious flaws. First, it eliminates the majority of people who get sick through gluten but do not display any tissue damage (I will present you with solid evidence for this in Chapter 6). Second, in the past, you had to be quite sick before a biopsy would be performed. Similarly, nowadays not everyone who experiences reactions from gluten can have an endoscopy, due to funding constraints. Again, this reinforces the link between gluten damage and the gut, therefore people with gut-related symptoms are more likely to be investigated than those with skin- or brain-related symptoms. Third, great reliance is placed on the findings of biopsys, however results from this procedure have often been found to be unreliable.

I am frequently asked whether it is possible to diagnose coeliac disease without having a small bowel biopsy. Similarly, I am commonly asked if the small bowel biopsy is the 'gold standard' for the diagnosis of coeliac disease. The answer to these questions is complex, and involves both semantics and changing knowledge about the ways in which gluten causes damage in the body.

Is there a 'gold standard'?

Is there currently a gold standard for the diagnosis of coeliac disease? The concept of a 'gold standard' comes from the monetary system. In the past, the standard economic unit of account was a fixed weight of gold – literally the 'gold standard'. This was supposed to remove 'currency uncertainty', however the world has long since abandoned the gold standard in favour of a more flexible system.

This 'gold standard' metaphor has been carried over into medicine however, where it has the connotation of an absolute benchmark in terms of diagnosis. Current medical dogma states that you can only make a diagnosis of coeliac disease if the small bowel biopsy shows villous atrophy. Hence the biopsy is seen as the 'gold standard' diagnostic test for coeliac disease.

However, this was based on a circular argument: coeliac disease was a flat biopsy, and a flat biopsy meant coeliac disease. Over the last few years, this notion of a 'gold standard' has been gradually undermined.

Histology uncertainty

There are problems with the interpretation of the histology of the small bowel in relation to coeliac disease. Marsh (1992) first suggested the application of criteria to grade the various degrees of histological damage. This was because the extent of the small intestinal changes can vary from normal mucosa with increase in intraepithelial lymphocytes (IEL) to a completely flat-looking mucosa. Subsequently, a group of pathologists revised Marsh's criteria and wrote a report seeking to standardize the histological features of coeliac disease and outlining a proposed reporting range. This is called the modified Marsh classification (Oberhuber et al, 1999):

Marsh score	IEL*	Crypts	Villi
Type 0	<40	Normal	Normal
Type 1	>40	Normal	Normal
Type 2	>40	Hypertrophic	Normal
Type 3a	>40	Hypertrophic	Mildatrophy
Type 3b	>40	Hypertrophic	Marked atrophy
Type 3c	>40	Hypertrophic	Total atrophy (flat)

* Numbers are given as intraepithelial lymphocytes/100 epithelial cells

Type 0 is normal small bowel tissue, however even these subjects could be reacting to gluten in their other organs. This demonstrates that a test of the gut for any abnormalities caused by gluten does not necessarily give a definitive yes/no answer. There is a spectrum of damage that needs to be interpreted within the overall context of clinical observation and the results of blood tests.

Type 3 (a, b & c) indicates villous atrophy of varying degrees (the word 'atrophy' means poorly growth or damage). The crypts are hypertrophic, which means overgrown because they are attempting to replace the cells being destroyed in the villi.

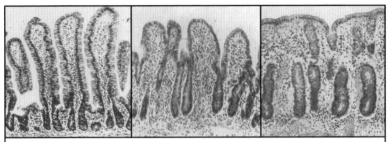

These three pictures are from small bowel biopsies of people investigated for coeliac disease. The first is an example of a *normal* small bowel biopsy, Type 0 (it shows the long finger-like villi and the crypt structure). The other two show abnormal mucosa with shortened villi and deepened crypts. They show *subtotal villus atrophy*, Type 3b, and *total villus atrophy*, Type 3c.

Types 1 & 2, situated between the extremes, suggest more subtle and/or early changes.

The question is, therefore: "Where do you draw the line regarding the characterization of small bowel damage in coeliac disease?"

Patchy histology makes sample unreliable

Another problem is that coeliac disease tends to be a patchy condition. The gluten damage is not uniform throughout the gut. Villous atrophy, the hallmark of coeliac disease, is patchy in the duodenum (Lee et al., 2005). This is another factor that makes the biopsy of the small bowel unreliable. Random biopsy, even of normal-appearing mucosa, is necessary for the diagnosis of coeliac disease. Thus at least four to six biopsy pieces need to be taken and examined. However, biopsy of the descending duodenum is sufficient. Going further down the bowel, even just a little, has been found to further increase the variability of the histology. Lee and his colleagues conclude that "Although characteristic endoscopic features may be useful, their absence does not exclude coeliac disease."

This finding is similar to that of an earlier study (Bonamico et al., 2004) demonstrating that children with coeliac disease may have patchy villous atrophy of the duodenum. The bulb mucosa may be the only duodenal area involved, both at diagnosis and after gluten challenge. Therefore, the authors recommend, multiple endoscopic biopsies should always be performed – not only in the distal duodenum, but also in the bulb.

Electron microscope shows up damage

Gluten sensitivity has been shown to be associated with 'minimal' mucosal changes, which cannot be seen with conventional light microscopy (Sarbati et al., 2003). In other words, tissue that appears normal under a standard microscope can be seen to be damaged under a more powerful machine.

For their study, duodenal biopsies of seven subjects with positive anti-endomysial antibodies (EMA) and apparently normal histology (using conventional microscopy) underwent 'ultrastructural' evaluation of the epithelial surface using electron microscopy. In four patients, the electron microscope revealed changes of the enterocyte brush border, with a significant reduction in the height of microvilli.

These patients were kept on gluten and after several months three of them had a second biopsy which showed histological changes suggestive of coeliac disease. The study concluded that "Such lesions, which primarily involve microvillous structure, may imply a reduction of intestinal absorptive surface that is already in the latent stage of the disease process."

Experienced pathologists needed

As you can see, this area of small bowel histology is complex. Not surprisingly, it has also been found that community histologists are less likely to pick up small bowel changes compared with histologists who specialize in the gut.

To conclude, it is clear that there can be no such thing as a 'gold standard' for the diagnosis of coeliac disease – the absolute reliability of the biopsy has been tarnished. Logically therefore, it follows that the diagnosis of coeliac disease should not hinge on the biopsy results alone. And so we turn to blood tests, however as you will see, the blood tests that are now available make things even more complicated!

You cannot rely on biopsy results

The blood test investigations

Take another look at the diagram showing the history of coeliac disease, in particular the third column, which indicates when blood tests were first used. As you can see, it was only in 1990, less than 20 years ago, that gluten reactivity in the body could first be detected by a blood test. Fortunately, antibody technology has progressed a lot since then, and this has precipitated enormous changes in the understanding of gluten sensitivity, yet again questioning the primacy of the small bowel biopsy result. There are two quite distinct types of blood test, each of which measure different phenomena: **gluten** tests; and **tissue damage** tests.

The gluten tests

Gluten is a protein that is found in wheat grains (you will learn all about gluten in the next chapter). This protein has a number of components, one of which is called **gliadin**. It so happens that the people who get sick from gluten are reacting to the gliadin component.

To understand what the blood tests mean, first you need to know a little more about your immune system. It is the job of your immune system to protect you from the outside world. It protects you from the invasion of microbes (viruses and bacteria), and it also protects you from the toxins and poisons in the food that passes through your gut.

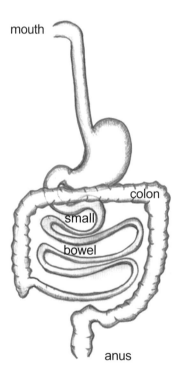

From this diagram, you can see that you have a long tube inside you that travels from your mouth to your anus. This is your gastrointestinal tract, also called your gut or your bowel.

Even though it is inside your body, the contents of this tube are still on the 'outside' from your body's point of view.

Lots of your immune cells coat the skin (called the mucosa) of this tube and work hard to protect you from anything that might prove to be harmful.

Gliadin attack

Gliadin, the toxic component of the gluten protein, is one such harmful substance. Your immune system defends your body strongly against gliadin using weapons called **antibodies** and the gliadin is repelled. The outcome of your immune system's fight against gliadin is the production of antibodies that are specifically targeted towards gliadin: these are called anti-gliadin antibodies.

Anti-gliadin antibodies (sometimes abbreviated to AGA) are weapons that have been made specifically to fight against gluten in the diet. Remember, gliadin is a component of the gluten protein.

There are two classes of gliadin antibodies: IgG-gliadin and IgA-gliadin. These antibodies are very sensitive. They are made very specifically by your immune system to fight against gliadin, however a high level of these antibodies does not necessarily mean that you have any gut damage, so they are not very accurate in assisting the identification of patients with histological small bowel damage.

High IgG-gliadin antibodies indicate a gluten reaction

Tests for these antibodies are nearly always strongly positive in people with coeliac disease who are not on a gluten-free diet. Once people are placed on a strict diet, these antibodies will fall to normal levels within a period of a few months to a year or two.

What does a high gliadin IgG antibody mean?

A high level of IgG-gliadin indicates that there has been a specific immune reaction to gluten in your body. It can be interpreted in one of four ways:

1)   In people *with* symptoms, it most commonly indicates a *gluten-sensitivity*. That is, being unwell because you are eating gluten in your diet.

2)   In *some* people *with* symptoms it indicates the early stages of coeliac disease, which can take many decades to develop. It is a valuable test for detecting people with 'potential coeliac disease'.

3)   In people *without* symptoms, it means that your immune system has been stimulated by the gliadin in your diet, but has not yet led to any health problems. For some, this is an early phase in the development of gluten-sensitivity. Others may never become unwell.

4)   In *some* people, a high IgG-gliadin level is associated with the gut damage caused by coeliac disease.

Levels of this antibody will become normal after 6–24 months of a gluten-free diet.

The gliadin IgA antibody

A high level of IgA-gliadin has a similar meaning to the IgG-gliadin antibody, however it is positive less often. If the level is elevated, the subject is very likely to have symptomatic gluten-sensitivity. IgA-gliadin does not become positive in everyone who has coeliac disease. This test can be useful for monitoring compliance with a gluten-free diet.

Levels of this antibody will also normalize after 6–24 months of a gluten-free diet.

The tissue damage markers

Coeliac disease is defined as the gut damage caused by gluten. When this occurs, there is an over-reaction of the immune system in the gut. A harmful immune reaction is generated in the gut mucosa. This tissue injury involves inflammatory cells and the production of antibodies.

The picture shows how small bowel tissue looks under the microscope. This is called the 'histology' of the tissue. The top frame shows the skin of *normal* upper bowel mucosa – you can see the long finger-like projections, called the villi (Marsh Type 0). Each black dot is a nucleus of a cell. The cells on the outside of the villi are responsible for the absorption of your food.

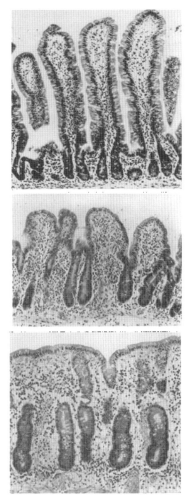

The middle panel shows what happens in established coeliac disease. The villi are damaged, and look short and poorly formed – this is an example of *partial villous atrophy* (Marsh Type 3b). By this stage there is an intense immune reaction occurring in these damaged tissues, including in the tiny muscles of the 'endomesium', that help keep the villi upright.

45

The bottom panel shows the havoc caused by long-standing coeliac disease – *total villous atrophy* or a 'flat' biopsy (Marsh Type 3c). As you can see, the damage is extreme.

ttG antibody

Damage to the endomysial muscle by gluten in the gut tissue stimulates the immune system to attack, and this produces the antibody **tissue transglutaminase (tTG)**. This is an antibody designed to defend against attacks on these tiny villous muscle tissues.

If you have high levels of tTG antibodies, this means that you could have gut damage from coeliac disease. An endoscopy will be required for confirmation.

The other tissue damage marker is the **endomysial antibody (EMA)**. Although it has the same sort of accuracy as the test used to measure the level of tTG antibodies, this is a more complicated test to carry out than the tTG test, therefore it is becoming less common.

ttG versus biopsy

Not surprisingly, research groups are now proposing that very high tTG levels indicate that patients are positive for coeliac disease, therefore they argue that a small bowel biopsy is not necessary for diagnosis for this select group (Barker et al., 2005). They suggest that in these circumstances a gluten-free diet should be commenced without a prior biopsy. However, others state that "All the other tests are only additional tests and cannot replace histology." Once again, this comes down to how coeliac disease is to be defined.

The coeliac HLA gene

There is great hope that the genetic marker for coeliac disease will be discovered in the not too distant future, however genetic testing for coeliac disease is currently imprecise.

It has been recently discovered that people with coeliac disease commonly have certain HLA genes (HLA is the 'histocompatibility leukocyte antigen'). It turns out that if you have type DQ2 or DQ8 HLA genes, then you have the genetic possibility of developing coeliac disease if you continue to eat gluten.

Carrying the type DQ2 and/or DQ8 HLA genes does not necessarily mean that you have, or are going to have coeliac disease, however it does mean that you carry a genetic susceptibility to suffering gut damage from gluten.

This gene is actually quite common. Population studies indicate that about 1 in 4 people (25%) have one of these genes, but only 1 in 100 people (1%) actually develop coeliac disease. This means that even if someone has the gene marker, there is only a 1 in 25 chance of having coeliac disease. Therefore, the presence of the coeliac gene is only indicative of the possibility of developing coeliac disease.

If your gene test is negative, it means that you are unlikely to develop coeliac disease (in a group of 100 coeliacs, only about 5 will not have the coeliac gene). However, a negative gene test does not protect you from gluten. This is about making the distinction between coeliac disease and *The Gluten Syndrome*. There are a multitude of symptoms caused by gluten which are not restricted to people with the coeliac gene (this will be covered in Chapter 4).

The HLA gene test is helpful in deciding who should go ahead and have a small bowel biopsy. If you do have the coeliac gene, there is no information available at this time to enable us to predict whether you might eventually develop coeliac disease, so it's important to keep yourself under surveillance, and repeat the blood tests every few years.

A note of caution on blood test results

The tissue tests for gut damage rely on your body being able to produce normal levels of immunoglobulin A. Therefore, these tests that measure IgA-based antibodies are of no value if the person has an IgA deficiency, a condition which is seen in about 10% of coeliacs.

The conflict of the IgG-gliadin test

There is a degree of conflict surrounding the interpretation of the gliadin antibody test, which indicates elevated levels in about 10% of the population.

To summarise, beginning in the 1990s, the anti-gliadin IgG antibody test (referred to as the IgG-gliadin test) was used to verify suspicion of coeliac disease, however it has been found to be a poor predictor of coeliac disease. In contrast, antibodies that are triggered by bowel tissue damage, namely the tissue transglutaminase (tTG) antibody and endomesial antibody (EMA), are excellent predictors of coeliac disease. Studies demonstrate that where levels of these antibodies are elevated, more than 95% of patients will be found to have coeliac disease. Not surprisingly, there are now claims that a high tTG level is all that is required to make a diagnosis of coeliac disease.

Equally unsurprisingly, there are two opposing schools of thought here. The medical establishment, represented by the gastroenterologists, has concluded that the gluten blood tests are inaccurate and misleading. They prefer to focus on the gut damage, and have shown that the gluten blood tests are poor in predicting who has the tissue damage caused by coeliac disease.

Further, they say that the gluten tests have poor sensitivity in detecting coeliac disease. All this is true, however they then go on to make an error of logic. They say that because the gluten tests are not useful in detecting coeliac disease, the gluten tests are not good for anything, and should therefore be abandoned.

The IgG-gliadin test is a gluten test

The counter-argument is that the IgG-gliadin antibody test is a valuable means of detecting people who are reacting adversely to gluten. The relationship between patient complaints and high levels of gluten antibodies has not been widely investigated. My research has shown that high levels of gluten antibodies accurately predict a beneficial response to a gluten-free diet. The argument is that high IgG-gliadin antibody levels are indicative of an immunological reaction to gluten, which can manifest as significant poor health – *The Gluten Syndrome.*

What does a high tTG antibody mean?

There is a special enzyme that is present in muscle tissue called tissue transglutaminase. It seems that this enzyme can combine with gliadin. For some reason, this makes tTG more easily recognized by the body's immune system. tTG has been shown to be the antigen that is recognized by endomesial antibodies in people with coeliac disease.

Currently, a high level of tTG antibodies (which are IgA-based) is the most accurate *blood test* on which to base the diagnosis of coeliac disease. If you have a positive tTG antibody reading, there is about a 90% chance (but not 100%) that you will have an abnormal biopsy, with the tell-tale signs of coeliac disease.

These tTG antibodies were discovered in 1998 (Molberg et al., 1998) and tests for detection of tTG became commercially available from 2000. They have the same sensitivity and specificity as the endomysium antibody assay, however the tTG test is less costly and its results more reproducible than the EMA test.

tTG antibody levels generally become negative 9–24 months after starting a gluten-free diet.

The EMA (endomesial antibody)

The endomysium is the delicate tissue that surrounds and supports the tiny muscle fibres in the villi. The endomesial antibody (EMA) is also an IgA-based antibody.

EMA has been found to be an effective specific blood test for screening populations for coeliac disease. This test will generally return negative results following 12–24 months of a gluten-free diet.

3. Menaced by gluten

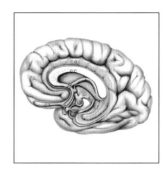

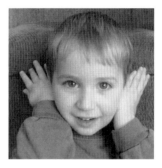

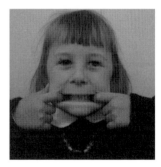

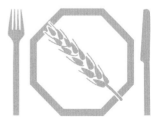

3. Menaced by gluten

Our planet struggles to feed the nearly eight billion people that crowd our world. The great plains of Europe, Asia and the Americas that are used to grow the mountains of grain that feed this hungry horde have been called the 'breadbaskets' of the world. These grains are laden with gluten; flour is made from these grains; bread is made from this flour; and gluten is making a lot of people unwell.

Gluten is sticky

You can't see gluten with your naked eye, but you can detect it by its properties, just as you can't see air, but you can detect its presence by feeling the wind on your face or compressing it in a bicycle pump.

The main property of gluten is its stickiness. Gluten is a complex protein that is formed by the combination of glutenin and gliadin as they get mixed together with water. Dough is gluey because of the gluten it contains. When you make dough with wheat-flour, it sticks to your hands because of the gluten. It is this property of stickiness that makes gluten so valuable in baking. It helps stick the food together, and gives a pleasing texture to the baked items. Wheat gluten is unique in its ability to form a sticky dough and thus produce a loaf of bread. Proteins from other sources, even at high levels, do not have this quality.

A kernel of wheat

A grain, or kernel, of wheat is composed of about 70% starch sugar and 30% protein. Starch is present only in the endosperm, but the protein is distributed through all parts of the grain. The components of gluten, gliadin and glutenin, also mostly come from the inside endosperm.

The wheat kernel, or grain of wheat, contains three distinct parts that are separated during the milling process to produce flour. About 10% of the kernel is protein. The endosperm is the store of food for the growing plant until it is able to draw nutrients form the outside environment.

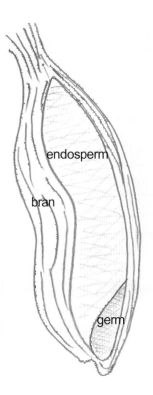

The 'endosperm' is the white floury filling inside the grain. It contains about 80% of the kernel weight. It contains the greatest proportion of the protein, particular the gluten.

The 'bran' is the tough outer skin that protects the grain while it is in the soil. It contains about 15% of the kernel weight. It contains only a small amount of protein.

The 'germ' is about 3% of the kernel. It is the sprouting part of the seed. It is often separated from the flour during milling because of its high fat content (about 10%) which limits shelf life.

Gluten affects flour quality

The protein content of the flour affects the strength of the dough. The various wheat-flour types contain differing amounts of the gluten forming proteins, gliadin and glutenin. The quantity of the gluten in the flour increases as its protein content increases. The protein level determines the kind of baking results that are obtained. In yeast breads, a strong gluten framework is required, hence high-gluten flours are used.

High gluten improves bread

High protein content also gives the dough better fermentation endurance – this means it will not collapse if there are delays in getting it into the oven. However for cakes, if too much gluten is produced (caused by either the protein content or too much handling), it will result in a tough quality.

Protein content	Type of flour
8–10%	Cake flour
9–10%	Pastry flour
10–11.5%	All-purpose flour
11–13%	Bread flour
14% and up	High-gluten flour

Gluten-rich grains are valued by the bread industry because they give the dough better elasticity, and so there has been pressure on the agricultural sector to develop and harvest grains that have even higher gluten content. Our understanding of food technology and plant breeding programs has become increasingly sophisticated, and gluten-rich grains are now the norm.

How can gluten make you unwell?

Can eating bread really make you ill? Well, yes it can. Wheat contains gluten, and gluten is a potentially toxic substance to you. One of the problems with gluten is that we do not break it down very well in our intestine. Your gut cannot fully digest it, therefore fragments of gluten can easily be absorbed into your body in an unchanged form.

In turn, this sets up an immune reaction. Your body makes those antibody weapons against gluten, and this process can go on to damage your body's organs – and, I believe, your brain and nerve pathways (see Chapter 5).

Gluten is found in processed foods

Gluten is steadily invading the food chain. When you start to look for it, you find gluten everywhere! You can find it in most of your processed foods, in your body-care products, and in your medications and toothpaste. In our wheat-based societies most children, most adults and most of the elderly consume large amounts of wheat-based products at every meal every day, throughout their lives.

This means that most people have never experienced a gluten-free period in their lives, other than during their first six months of life. Therefore it's impossible for them to know whether gluten could be causing them harm. Tens of millions of people have been putting up with various symptoms all of their lives, and have simply got used to them. Even though they are perpetually unwell, they do not recognize that they are unwell. They think that they are 'normal', because being sick is the only experience that they know. They do not know the joy of good health.

Gluten overload

The amount of gluten in the Western diet continues to increase. Bread has become a staple food, and is seen as the base of 'the food pyramid'. The bottom of the pyramid consists of grains and breads, and the recommendation is for people to eat the highest proportion of their food from gluten-grains.

Fast-food outlets serve up meals on buns, on breads and on pizza bases, all made from gluten-laden flour. In addition, we are eating ever-bigger servings of gluten-laden foods. Wheat-based gluten foods are also relatively cheap. This makes these foods more attractive to people on low incomes. Globalisation of the food industry and aggressive advertising is narrowing the range of foods that people are able to choose from. There is a movement towards eating more foods that contain gluten and less fruits and vegetables.

Finally, gluten has been shown to be addictive. Gluten can behave in a similar way to morphine. We humans produce a morphine-like substance naturally in our own brains – these chemicals are called 'endorphins'. These endorphins are released in our brains to give us a sense of pleasure. They are also released in our brain as part of our body's natural mechanism to help numb pain. We can crave for the pleasure of this sensation.

Research now indicates that gluten can generate some of these pleasurable effects. This means that eating gluten can give you a real sense of pleasure, through stimulation of the morphine-like receptors in your brain. This explains why so many people seem to be addicted to wheat-based products. Cakes, dumplings, steamed puddings and big hunks of bread are often referred to as 'comfort foods'. For some people, the comfort is being derived from the morphine-like effect that the gluten is having on their brains.

4. The Gluten Syndrome

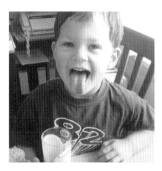

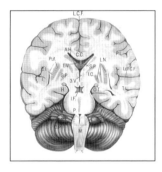

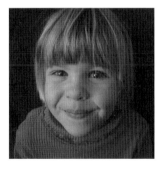

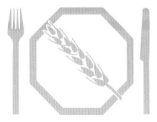

4. The Gluten Syndrome

Sick, tired or grumpy?

Are you feeling sick, tired or grumpy? If you are, then you might be suffering from *The Gluten Syndrome*. The symptoms can be subtle, but can interfere significantly with your lifestyle. These niggling symptoms, always feeling tired and irritable, serve to sap your energy.

The term *The Gluten Syndrome* applies to any reaction that is caused by gluten. This includes the myriad symptoms that are experienced throughout your gastro-intestinal tract. It also includes the host of other symptoms that do not stem from your gut. These include brain and behaviour disorders, irritability and tiredness, skin problems, muscle aches and pains, and joint problems. *The Gluten Syndrome* also includes the diagnosis of coeliac disease (the medical data on which this syndrome is based is presented in Chapters 5 and 6).

What's new?

So why is this syndrome new? Why has it been overlooked for so long? The reason is that there is no single recognizable illness that is caused by gluten. Also, the gluten blood tests, which you will recall were only developed in the 1990s, have helped to uncover the problem. There is a three-step process to finding out if you are affected by *The Gluten Syndrome*. The three steps are:
1.   Check out your symptoms
2.   Get your blood tests
3.   Interpret your results.

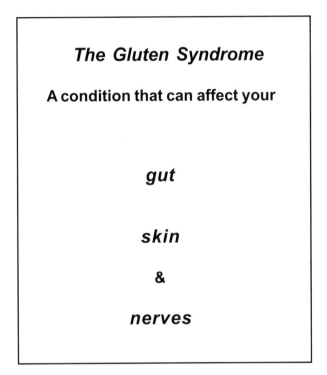

The Gluten Syndrome

A condition that can affect your

gut

skin

&

nerves

Check out your symptoms

Gluten reactions can trigger a wide range of symptoms and illnesses. Of course, gluten is not the cause of all our ailments, but it is responsible for many of the chronic aches and pains, and persistent mood and behaviour problems, that just don't go away.

Most people with *The Gluten Syndrome* have repeatedly sought help and advice from their medical services, but have not come away with a satisfactory answer. Their symptoms and health problems can be wide-ranging. It can involve your gut, your skin and your nerves.

These symptoms are listed on the next page. If you can answer 'yes' to any of these symptoms, you could be suffering from *The Gluten Syndrome*.

Many symptoms are caused by gluten

The Gluten Syndrome symptoms

Do you or your family have any of these problems?

- ☐ tired and exhausted
- ☐ uncomfortable tummy
- ☐ bloating and gas troubles
- ☐ gastric reflux or heartburn
- ☐ diarrhoea or constipation

- ☐ unhappy with your weight
- ☐ not growing well
- ☐ eating problems
- ☐ lack energy, weakness
- ☐ run-down

- ☐ runny nose and sinus problems
- ☐ chronic iron deficiency
- ☐ osteoporosis or growing pains
- ☐ dermatitis, eczema, itchy or bad skin
- ☐ infertility

- ☐ headaches or migraine
- ☐ feel depressed or moody or grumpy
- ☐ find it hard to think clearly
- ☐ poor sleep

- ☐ hyperactive or cranky
- ☐ Attention Deficit Hyperactivity Disorder (ADHD)
- ☐ autism
- ☐ mental health problems

If you can answer "yes" to any of these problems,
then you or your children could have *The Gluten Syndrome*.

The ten target areas

The diagram of the ten target areas in the diagram puts these symptoms in context. These are the ten areas in your body that can be adversely affected by gluten. Each target area is indicated by a diamond-shaped box. As you can see, the small bowel (the focus of coeliac disease) is only one of these target areas. In this scheme, coeliac disease is included as part of *The Gluten Syndrome*. The ten target areas are:

Gut related symptoms
1. Mouth   – ulcers, runny nose, sore throat.
2. Oesophagus – gastro-oesophageal reflux, heart burn, swallowing difficulties.
3. Stomach   – indigestion, slow emptying, gastritis.
4. Small bowel – coeliac disease (enteropathy), malabsorption, diarrhoea.
5. Colon   – diarrhoea and constipation, bloating, low immune function.
6. Rectum   – constipation, soiling (encopresis).

Other symptoms
7. Brain   – disturbed behaviour, migraine, grumpy, tired, headache, depression, mood disorders, ataxia, autism, epilepsy, Attention Deficit Hyperactivity Disorder (ADHD).
8. Skin   – Dermatitis Herpetiformis, eczema.
9. Immune   – run-down, low immunity, recurrent infections.
10. Growth   – poor height and weight (short and/or thin).

Nutritional consequences

In addition to damage to these target areas, there are also the nutritional consequences of a poorly functioning gut. These problems include:

o   Bones and joints   – osteoporosis, bone and joint pain.
o   Nutritional deficiency – anaemia, osteoporosis, low levels of vitamins and minerals.
o   Infertility

Ten gluten-sensitive target areas

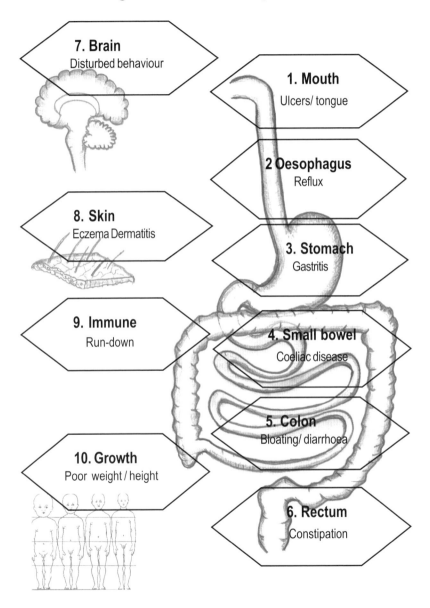

7. Brain
Disturbed behaviour

1. Mouth
Ulcers/ tongue

2 Oesophagus
Reflux

8. Skin
Eczema Dermatitis

3. Stomach
Gastritis

9. Immune
Run-down

4. Small bowel
Coeliac disease

5. Colon
Bloating/ diarrhoea

10. Growth
Poor weight / height

6. Rectum
Constipation

Get your blood tests

If you have symptoms that indicate you might have *The Gluten Syndrome*, I urge you to get some blood tests. Please do not go on a gluten-free diet until you have had your blood tests done. These blood tests will help you make a more accurate diagnosis and will guide you with your treatment. Also, your symptoms could be caused by something other than gluten. Therefore, you need to be properly investigated before you attribute your symptoms to gluten. Finally, it is important to detect whether you have any gut damage caused by coeliac disease.

So, please make sure that you get your blood tests. If you have been gluten-free for months or years, then it might be too late to get the blood tests. If you are in this situation, I have some advice for you later in this Chapter. These are the specific tests that I recommend:

❏   **ttG antibody** (also called IgA tissue transglutaminase) or **endomesial antibodies (EMA)**
❏   **IgG-gliadin** (also called IgG anti-gliadin antibody) This test is essential - ask if your lab can do this test.
❏   **IgA-gliadin** (also called IgA anti-gliadin antibody)
❏   **Total IgA antibody level** To look for deficiency of IgA antibody production.
❏   **Ferritin** to measure of your iron stores.
❏   **Hb** (Haemoglobin) to check for anaemia.
❏   **CRP** (C-Reactive protein) to look for inflammation.
❏   and **DGP** (Deamidated Gliadin Peptide) a new test.

The reasons for getting these blood tests are as follows:

ttG antibody (also called IgA tissue transglutaminase antibody)
The ttG antibody test is a tissue damage test. ttG is a specific antibody made against muscle tissue damage in your small bowel. It is a very sensitive indicator of the small bowel damage

that can be caused by the gluten in your diet. High levels of ttG mean that you might have gut damage (coeliac disease). It is currently recommended that you confirm the likelihood of gut damage by having a small bowel biopsy (by endoscopy).

IgG-gliadin (also called IgG anti-gliadin antibody)

IgG-gliadin antibody is a gluten reaction test. IgG-gliadin is a specific antibody made by your immune system when it is assaulted by the gluten that you eat in your diet. A raised level of IgG-gliadin indicates that you have an *immunological* response to gluten, and tells you that you might be getting symptoms from gluten. This is the most reliable blood test for gluten-sensitivity, and high levels are also associated with coeliac disease. In my experience, the majority of people with high IgG-gliadin levels have *The Gluten Syndrome,* but most do not have coeliac disease.

Importantly, not all laboratories do the same test. Different 'antibody kits' are used that give varying responses. My experience of the IgG-gliadin tests in my patients is based on the test systems of *Inova Diagnostics*, San Diego, USA.

DGP (Deamidated Gliadin Peptide)

This is a new type of gliadin test is being manufactured by *Inova Diagnostics*. It has been developed to more accurately identify people with coeliac disease. Eventually, it is likely to overtake the ttG test because it is excellent at finding those people who have gluten gut damage. This test detects an immune response to a very specific fragment of the gluten molecule (this fragment is a short peptide of gliadin). This new test is excellent for detecting coeliac disease (in fact it seems more reliable that the ttG test), but it will not detect gluten sensitivity in people who do not have coeliac disease. It will not pick up the people who have the other symptoms of *The Gluten Syndrome*. It does not replace the IgG-gliadin test.

IgA-gliadin (also called IgA anti-gliadin antibody)

IgA-gliadin antibody is also a gluten test. IgA-gliadin is a specific antibody made against gluten, but an IgA class antibody which is made by immune cells situated in the gut mucosa. A high level of this IgA-gliadin antibody indicates that you are generating an strong immunological response to the gluten in your diet. High levels are frequently associated with coeliac disease. Most people with a high IgA-gliadin antibody test result are gluten-sensitive and have *The Gluten Syndrome.*

Total IgA antibody levels

This is looking for any deficiency in your IgA antibody production. The total IgA antibody level is a measurement of the IgA class of antibody, which is frequently low in people with gluten-sensitivity and coeliac disease. There are two reasons for measuring total IgA. First, if the level of total IgA is low, or absent, it makes the tTG result invalid (because tTG is an IgA-based antibody). Second, low total IgA immunoglobulins make gluten-sensitivity a more likely diagnosis.

Ferritin

This is a measure of your iron stores. People who react to gluten are frequently deficient in iron. The serum ferritin is a useful measurement of your iron stores. If levels are low, an iron supplement should be taken to get your iron levels back to normal. Low iron stores are associated with irritability, tiredness and low immune status. If you have *The Gluten Syndrome*, then your gut may not be absorbing iron very well.

Hb (Haemoglobin)

This is to check for anaemia. Your haemoglobin measures the oxygen-carrying capacity of your blood. Low iron levels will cause your Hb to fall, and if your iron levels get too low, you will become anaemic. Other nutritional deficiencies can also lead to anaemia. People who are gluten-sensitive are frequently iron deficient.

CRP (C-Reactive protein)
This is to look for evidence of inflammation. CRP is an inflammatory marker. If you are unwell with an infection, then this test will be high. A high level of CRP will invalidate the serum ferritin levels. Also, an underlying inflammation might point to something else being wrong with you.

In addition, several other blood tests should also be considered, depending on your overall health, age and symptoms:

HLA DQ2/DQ8
To determine whether you have the genetic predisposition for coeliac disease (see Chapter 2)

Thyroid function
Thyroid problems are associated with gluten problems

Blood sugar
Diabetes is a common problem that causes many people to feel sick, tired and grumpy

Vitamin levels (D, folate, B12)
Poor absorption of vitamins is another clue to why you might be unwell. People with poor gut function often have nutritional deficiencies.

Liver function
Liver dysfunction is associated with gluten reactions

Total IgE levels
Gives an indication of overall allergic status.

As you can see, there are a lot of things that can go wrong. The more you investigate, the better your diagnosis is likely to be, the better your treatment, and consequently the better your prognosis.

Interpret your results

Your third step is to get an accurate interpretation of your blood tests. In my opinion, the results of these tests are often misinterpreted. In particular, the IgG-gliadin levels are frequently dismissed as being 'non-specific' or even meaningless. However, my research shows that the IgG-gliadin levels are a crucial measurement, and support the diagnosis of gluten-sensitivity.

I suggest that you obtain the actual results (together with the normal ranges) of your blood tests. You will then be able to use the following flow charts to help you interpret your results. There are two charts: one for those with a positive tTG result, and a second chart for those with a negative tTG result. I will take you through these charts, step by step.

If you have positive tTG result

Use **Flow chart 1** if you have a positive tTG result. This initial decision is based upon the tTG result because it can identify whether you might have coeliac disease. Although a high tTG suggests the presence of coeliac disease, an endoscopy is still recommended to provide confirmation. This procedure looks for any small bowel damage (villous atrophy). A confirmed diagnosis of coeliac disease is important, because it means that you will then be committed to a life-long gluten-free diet. Coeliac disease diagnosis carries other implications, including the need to search for it in other family members.

Part of your investigations might include looking at your HLA DQ2/DQ8 genetic marker for coeliac disease. If this is positive, then you have an increased chance of having coeliac disease. This test can be used to help make a decision about who might warrant an endoscopy.

Flow-chart 1

How to interpret your blood test results if **ttG** is **positive**

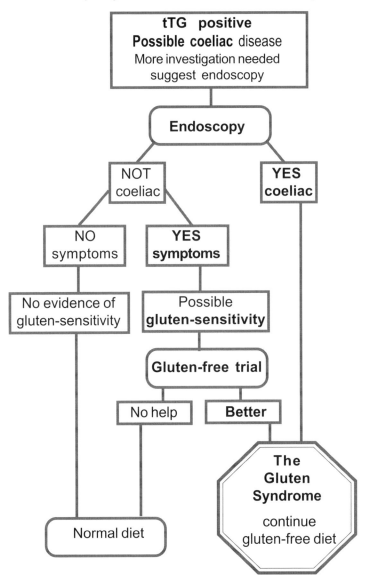

If your endoscopy is normal (about a third of people with a high tTG will have a normal endoscopy, especially children), *and* if you have symptoms, *and* if your IgG-gliadin antibody is high, then your next step is to trial a gluten-free diet for a few months. If you feel better at the end of this trial, you will know that you have *The Gluten Syndrome*.

If you have negative tTG result

Use **Flow chart 2** if you have a negative tTG result. With a low tTG, it is unlikely that you have coeliac disease, but there are some exceptions to this statement. You have to make sure that your total IgA level is normal (a low total IgA level invalidates the tTG result). Also, in children, especially those under five years of age, the tTG result can be misleading (coeliac disease is a progressive disease – it comes on slowly, so early in the disease there may not be enough gut damage to cause the tTG antibody levels to rise). If there is sufficient clinical evidence to arouse suspicion of coeliac disease, then go ahead with an endoscopy.

The decision point in this chart depends on your gliadin (IgG or IgA) antibodies. A high gliadin antibody level is evidence that your immune system is reacting to gluten. Population studies show that about 10% of people have a raised IgG-gliadin level. If you have symptoms, then you are probably gluten-sensitive (but free of coeliac disease). The final step is to try a gluten-free diet for a few months. If you feel better at the end of this period, then it is clear that you have *The Gluten Syndrome*.

It is worth noting that a number of people react to gluten even though they have normal levels of gliadin antibodies. This means that if you have symptoms that suggest you are gluten-sensitive, then you have nothing to lose by trying a gluten-free diet. Again, if you begin to feel better, then you have *The Gluten Syndrome*.

Flow-chart 2

How to interpret your blood test results if **tTG** is **negative**

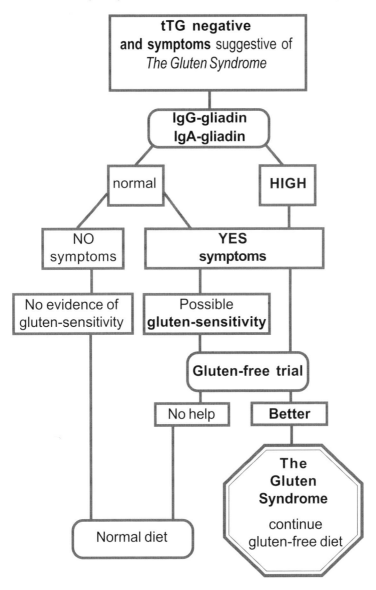

Help from the Doctor Gluten website

If you have followed the flow sheets but still would like some help with the interpretation of your blood tests, then follow these steps:

1. Get your results.
2. Go to **www.doctorgluten.com**
3. Enter your test results at **Blood Test Results**
   (http://www.doctorgluten.com/bloodresults.htm)
4. You will then be sent an interpretation of your blood test results with suggestions as to what action you should take.

If you did not get a blood test

One of the most common questions I am asked is, "I am already on a gluten-free diet – can I still have a blood test?" Another common question is, "Do I need to go back on to gluten to get my blood tests?"

Gluten-free for less than a year

The blood tests for gluten take about six months or more to show changes once you go gluten-free. So, if you have been gluten-free for only a few weeks or months, then it is still okay to get your blood tests done without going back on gluten. But make sure that you get all the blood tests that you need – see the blood tests list a few pages back for details. These blood tests measure the immune reaction to gluten (the IgG-gliadin antibodies) and give an indication of any gut damage (the tTG antibody).

These antibodies are being produced all the time by your immune system. They are manufactured by your immune cells in response to gluten attack. It takes months for these immune cells to stop producing these antibodies, so your blood tests can be done any time up to 6 or 12 months after you go on a gluten-free diet. There is no need to go back on to gluten prior to the blood tests, as long as it has only been a few months, or a year at most, since you started on a gluten-free diet.

This does not apply to the small bowel biopsy, done by endoscopy. That test needs you to be on gluten at the time of testing. This is because the gut damage usually heals within a month of going gluten-free.

Gluten-free for more than a year
If you have been on a gluten-free diet for more than a year, your antibody levels for both gliadin and tTG may have been lowered to normal levels. Therefore, your blood test will give you an accurate reflection of your (largely overcome) illness, however the quest for a blood test is often driven by the need to obtain a 'formal' diagnosis. For instance, I received this note from Kate:

> "I have cut out gluten from my diet and feel remarkably better off for doing so. I have been off gluten for nearly two years now, however I want to get the blood testing done to officially 'confirm or deny' whether I am in fact intolerant to gluten. How long do I need to re-include gluten in my diet before I can go and get my blood tests done and be confident of an accurate result? Any advice you can give me would be appreciated."

There are several strands to answering this question.
1 – This hinges on the difference between coeliac disease and gluten-sensitivity. For most medical practitioners, coeliac disease is currently the only 'official' medical diagnosis for gluten reactions, and in order for them to be able to formally make this diagnosis, you need to be on gluten, test positive to the tissue damage antibody tests (tTG or EMA) and have a positive small bowel biopsy. About 1 in 100 people have coeliac disease.

2 – The gluten-sensitivity diagnosis can be made by looking at both the levels of gluten antibodies and your clinical response to going on a gluten-free diet. As you feel heaps better when you are off gluten, it stands to reason that you are gluten-sensitive (you had a good clinical response to going gluten-free).

3 – As you have been off gluten for over a year, then the blood tests will show normal levels, so it is a waste of time doing them. You can try going back on gluten for a few weeks and then getting tested. This will stimulate your immune cells to produce the gluten antibodies again. Understand though that you are also likely to feel unwell again. That will be a good test for you to confirm whether you still get symptoms with gluten in your diet.

4 – The bottom line is, if you feel a lot better when you're off gluten, then it's best for you to stay off gluten and enjoy your new found health. You have *The Gluten Syndrome,* but fortunately, you also have the answer to your troubles.

Going gluten free

By now, you have heard a lot about gluten, and probably realize that you might need to go on a gluten-free diet. So what is a gluten-free diet? We have written a whole book on this called *Going gluten-free: how to get started,* however here I give you a brief summary of the main points.

What foods do I avoid?

Going gluten-free means avoiding all foods that contain gluten. Gluten is one of the many proteins found in the following three grains:

o wheat
o barley
o rye.

What about oats?

What about oats, I hear you ask? There has been controversy for years as to whether or not it is okay to eat oats if you are gluten-sensitive. Oats do not contain gluten, but can be contaminated in harvesting and processing. Some people are intolerant to both oats and gluten. Put simply, a gluten-free diet means avoiding all foods that contain wheat, rye, barley and, possibly, oats.

However it's not that easy. Gluten is a useful ingredient in the manufacturing and processing of many foods, therefore you may well find that gluten has been added to food that has been refined and processed, regardless of whether it contains wheat, rye, barley or oats. Anything that comes in a packet could contain some gluten.

What food can I eat?

Before you get too dispirited, let's look at the foods that you can eat! This is a short but complete list of unprocessed foods which are gluten-free:

o   All fruits
o   All vegetables, legumes, beans
o   All meats, fish, poultry, eggs
o   All simple dairy products
o   All gluten-free cereals
o   All nuts.

The significance of the qualifiers 'unprocessed' and 'simple' is that during processing, manufacturers frequently add gluten-containing substances. This is for reasons related to food technology. Likewise, processed organic foods may also contain gluten. Unfortunately, gluten is a very useful ingredient in food manufacturing processes. Meat, chicken, fish, rice, fruits and vegetables do not contain gluten, so you can eat as much of these foods as you like.

Gluten-free is easy

Starting on a gluten-free diet might seem daunting at first, but once you understand where gluten is found, it becomes easy. With time, identifying sources of gluten will become second nature to you. You will soon know which foods are safe and which are not. Within a few weeks, you will be an expert.

Once you try – it becomes easy

Despite the gluten restrictions, you can still eat a well-balanced diet that includes a variety of foods. There are also excellent gluten-free breads and pasta substitutes. For example, instead of wheat flour, you can use flours made from potato, rice, soy or beans.

No need for gluten

There is no biological need for you to eat gluten. Gluten does not have any health-giving properties. A life without gluten is a healthy lifestyle. You will begin to explore using amaranth, arrowroot, buckwheat, chick pea, millet and tapioca.

Being gluten-free is not about limiting your diet, rather it is about expanding the variety of foods that you eat. Most people, when asked about their gluten-free diet, say that they are eating healthier and better than they have ever done before.

Many food additives contain gluten

The great masquerader

Coeliac disease has been likened to a chameleon, in that it keeps on changing its appearance. Over the hundred years during which it has been under scrutiny, coeliac disease has changed from a clinical description of poor growth and diarrhoea to what is now a catalogue of symptoms of an illness.

Coeliac disease has been called the great masquerader, because people with established coeliac disease can have extremely varied symptoms and other associated diseases. The manifestations of coeliac disease extend far beyond damage to the tissue of the small bowel. The medical literature is full of descriptions of disorders that have been shown to be related to the presence of coeliac disease. The conundrum is that these other disorders may not provide any apparent clinical clue, indeed they may even mask the fact, that there is underlying coeliac disease.

A list of these related conditions follows on the next two pages. I have placed the neurological conditions at the top of the list, as I think that neurological damage is the primary mechanism of the gluten reaction.

Yes, there are many disorders related to the presence of coeliac disease. This is part of *The Gluten Syndrome* which especially affects your gut, your skin and your nerves.

A multitude of symptoms are caused by gluten

Associated disorders related to the presence of coeliac disease

Brains and nerves

Peripheral neuropathy and myopathy
Epilepsy, convulsions
Ataxia
Myelopathy
Psychiatric disturbances
Depression and mood disorders

Mouth and gut

Recurrent aphthous mouth ulcers
Defects in tooth enamel
Pharyngeal and oesophageal carcinoma
Reflux oesophagitis
Lymphocytic gastritis
Liver disease
Irritable bowel syndrome
Ulcerative jejunitis
Adenocarcinoma of small bowel

Hormones

Type 1 diabetes
Infertility in men and women
Recurrent abortion
Thyroid disorders
Adrenal disorders (Addison's disease)

Blood and immune

Anaemia (iron, folate and vitamin B12 deficiency)
Coagulation disorders from vitamin K deficiency
IgA deficiency
Hyposplenism
T-cell lymphoma
Cardiomyopathy

Bones and joints

Osteopenia
Arthralgia/arthritis
Osteoporosis
Growing pains

Skin and hair

Dermatitis herpetiformis
Eczema
Psoriasis
Brown pigmentation of face and cheek mucosa
Alopecia areata (hair loss)

Genetic

Trisomy 21 (Down's syndrome)

Gluten-sensitivity can cause all of these problems

Gluten is the culprit

This is an extraordinary list of complaints, all of which have been associated with coeliac disease. The question that has not been addressed is, what can possibly cause all of these symptoms. It seems implausible that some patchy intestinal damage could be responsible for such a wide range of symptoms and illnesses. It also seems unlikely that this list can be explained away by nutritional deficiencies.

Undoubtedly, some of these symptoms are due to gut damage and malnutrition, but not all of them. So, what can be the explanation?

One in ten are affected by gluten

My hypothesis, well-supported by the medical literature, is that it is gluten that causes these symptoms, by upsetting the neurological system. Gluten causes a malfunction of the brain and nervous networks throughout the body. In particular, the autonomic nervous system becomes dysfunctional. This process is fully documented in my book *Full of it! The shocking truth about gluten.*

5. Gluten upsets your nerves and brain

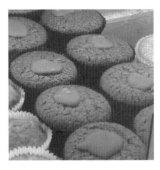

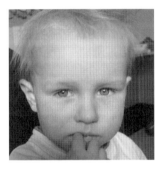

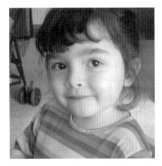

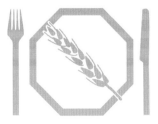

5. Gluten upsets your nerves and brain

The Gluten Syndrome is a sickness of your nerves and brain. I have come to this conclusion after studying the effects of gluten on my patients for over a decade. I am a paediatric gastroenterologist and allergist, and I run a clinic for children and their parents. Over the years I had become increasingly concerned by the large numbers of patients I was seeing who were affected by gluten.

I was perplexed by their wide-ranging symptoms. The puzzle was to explain how gluten could cause some much ill-health for so many people in so many different ways. This included coeliac disease, but I was certain that these symptoms could not all be attributed to just gut damage.

How does gluten cause so much harm?

I pondered the questions "Why do they have such an array of symptoms from gluten?", "Why do they recover so quickly when gluten is removed?" and "Why do they deteriorate so rapidly when only tiny amounts of gluten are eaten?" The concept of a brain/nerve disease can explain everything. I therefore postulate that gluten can damage your brain.

Faulty brain control

Eureka! The likely solution to this problem came when I was deep in discussion with my friend and colleague Ron Harper, Professor of Neurobiology at the University of California in Los Angeles. We were both struggling with the concept of multiple symptoms that needed to be explained by a single mechanism.

The answer was absurdly simple: disturbed 'brain control'. It suddenly seemed obvious – gluten was disturbing the neural pathways of the body. That provided one source that would explain all the symptoms. We wondered if gluten could be gradually damaging the brain and the nerves of susceptible people. Maybe it was the brain that was the common pathway for the manifestations of all the various gluten symptoms. The next step was to research the medical literature.

Is gluten a neurotoxin?

I felt excited, and commenced reviewing my patients in this new light. I began to see gluten as a neurotoxin – this could provide a universal model of gluten-sensitivity and would explain *The Gluten Syndrome*. I was looking for a 'brain-grain' connection.

The medical literature suggested that this toxicity might act through inflammatory mechanisms or cross-reactivity with neurons. The evidence was accumulating in support of my proposal that gluten-sensitivity was a brain and nerve disease.

Gluten causes damage through brain and nerves

Food allergy sceptics

I have an enquiring mind, and so I am always questioning the information that I am taught. As a junior doctor, I decided to conduct formal research into the food allergy phenomenon. This was because I was seeing children in hospital who seemed to get sick when they were fed milk or eggs, however my colleagues did not agree with me, and were sceptical towards my theory. At that time, there were articles being published in the medical journals with titles such as *Food allergy – fact or fiction?*

I was successful in obtaining a two-year research post and proceeded to carry out the first comprehensive food allergy studies ever done in New Zealand using the randomised double-blind control trial method that is considered the benchmark of clinical research.

I felt triumphant when, as a result of this research, I was able to demonstrate that food allergy was both real and common, but to my disappointment, my colleagues were reluctant to believe me or my data. They continued to express 'disbelief' towards the concept of food allergy.

This surprised me, as the results of the research I had presented had been obtained using strict scientific criteria. It was then that I began to realise that it might take more than hard data to change a person's belief system. Perhaps the thought of an adverse reaction to a food goes against the laws of nature in the minds of many people.

My next step was to do four more years of investigation into food allergy in Australia (at the Royal Children's Hospital in Melbourne). This was a bigger and more elaborate study. My doctoral thesis based on this work was titled *Food hypersensitivity in children: diagnostic approaches to milk and egg hypersensitivity* (1982).

Since then, I have continued my investigations into food allergy, yet today, 25 years on, medical scepticism continues to abound. This 'disbelief' is maintained despite the vast amount of research now available describing food allergy. There seems to be an underlying unwillingness on the part of doctors to consider food allergy as a possibility. Unfortunately, this now also applies to gluten reactions.

Medics turn a blind eye

Disturbingly, gluten is causing tremendous damage but, currently, this is mostly going unrecognised. Gluten grains have become our staple diet, thus the quantity of gluten in our food has been steadily increasing. Even worse, official health policies endorse gluten grains as the foundation of our food pyramid.

Because we are eating stacks of gluten-carrying breads and other products, gluten is sapping the energy and wellbeing of countless millions of people. To date, the medical profession has turned a blind eye to the wider range of problems caused by gluten while focusing their attention solely on coeliac disease.

A typical gluten story

I receive thousands of emails such as this:
"Dr Ford, I have emailed you a number of times regarding our two children. I thought I should let you know that since going gluten-free for the last three months, our son and daughter have put on some weight at last.

If I had kept them on a normal gluten diet (which they recommended at the hospital) we would still be having the headaches and sore tummies, as well as the bad moods which our son was experiencing. People just thought he was a naughty child, but now he is so different – we can talk to him without getting into any fights.

I congratulate you for all your efforts on bringing gluten intolerance to the attention of the media and the medical profession. More children and their families may find long-awaited relief. We have had to put up with this for seven years! At long last, there is light at the end of the tunnel. Kind regards, Sue and Garry."

Can gluten damage your brain?

I believe that gluten was making Sue and Garry's two children sick. That was the reason for their 'naughty' behaviour, their moods and their headaches.

The brain/nerve hypothesis states that *"The Gluten Syndrome occurs through gluten's action on the nervous system."* I propose that gluten-sensitivity is a brain condition.

Each and every organ in your body is in some way under the influence of brain/nerve control. I propose that gluten can injure the delicate nervous networks that control your gut's functions. A malfunction will subsequently lead to all of the gut symptoms that have been so well described. In addition, gluten can also directly affect brain function, which leads to the primary neurological symptoms that are so commonly seen with gluten-sensitivity. This gives a unifying theory to the symptoms that are attributed to gluten toxicity.

Tariq's gluten story

His mother wrote to me saying:

"Dear Rodney,

Thank you for your care and support of my family in regard to our allergies, gluten-sensitivity and coeliac disease.

My son Tariq, who is nearly 12 years old, has been a patient of yours for a number of years for his multiple food allergies. He also suffers from dyslexia. Over the last few years, Tariq had been becoming increasingly tired, lacking in energy and motivation, struggling with school work and constantly scratching due to the eczema and rashes that were covering all of his body.

During this time, even though he attended soccer training up to four times a week, he somehow gained a lot of weight. He was constantly grumpy, and had low mood levels.

Two months ago you diagnosed Tariq with gluten-sensitivity (his tTG was 4, IgG-gliadin 86 and IgA-gliadin 9).

Tariq was extremely reluctant to go on a gluten-free diet, but the rest of the family had gone gluten-free, so he was forced to become gluten-free along with the rest of us.

The changes that a gluten-free diet has evoked in Tariq have been astounding. His energy levels have increased, his skin has vastly improved, he has lost a lot of his excess weight (even though his appetite has increased) and he has shown improvement in his dyslexia.

Tariq is not as grumpy as he was, and his mood levels have improved. He is now vigilant about gluten and can see the differences it has made to the quality of his life.

The other soccer parents have also noticed a vast improvement in Tariq's energy levels and speed. His teacher has also noticed a big difference."

Thanks again.
Regards, Rosemary.

Your brain controls your gut

Your brain contains about 25 billion neurons, talking across more than 100 trillion synapses, along more than 100 million meters of nerve axons. This is an unbelievably vast neural network, and it is all contained within your skull and your spinal cord – just five kilograms of tissue. Amazing!

Perhaps even more astonishing is that you have a 'tummy brain'. This is another vast network of nerves that reaches to every part of your internal organs, and your 'tummy'. It has the same number of nerve cells and nerve fibres as the brain in your head. Your *head brain* and your *tummy brain* work together to process the food that you eat, however they each have some measure of independence.

Conscious and unconscious gut function

Brain function is traditionally sub-divided into 'conscious' and 'unconscious' activity. In relation to your gut, your brain has the following conscious activities:

o   Choice of what food you eat
o   Feeding yourself
o   Cerebral activity before eating (thinking about your food)
o   Smell, taste and texture
o   Chewing and swallowing
      … and, eventually …
o   Emptying your rectum (defecation).

Most of your gut function is unconscious. There is a big gap in your awareness of your gut between your mouth and your bottom end. While your food is being processed and digested, your brain is carrying out its unconscious activities. Hormone and enzyme production is also an important part of this phase.

The unconscious activity of your gut includes:

o   Peristalsis (the muscle activity that constantly moves your food along)
o   Oesophagal activity to move food from your mouth to your stomach
o   Stomach activity (acid and enzyme production and food grinding)
o   Small bowel (enzyme production and movement)
o   Gall bladder (making bile and contractions)
o   Pancreas (enzyme release)
o   Large bowel (movements and waste management)
o   Rectum (storage and dumping).

Gluten and the Autonomic Nervous System

Occam's razor (the law of succinctness) states that an explanation should make as few assumptions as possible. Defining *The Gluten Syndrome* as a neurological condition achieves this. It explains why there are so many and such varied manifestations of gluten-sensitivity, while making a minimal number of assumptions.

The proposition is that gluten injures the nerve networks that control gut function. In addition, gluten can also directly affect the brain, which leads to the primary neurological symptoms that are commonly seen with gluten-sensitivity.

The Autonomic Nervous System

How is all this unconscious gut activity achieved? It is your Autonomic Nervous System that gets the job done. This comprises all the nerves that interconnect between your internal organs: your gut, your heart and your glands.

This intricate network is shown in the diagram on the next page. Special 'control' nerves emerge from the spinal cord at each spinal level, between each vertebra. They are shown in the diagram as a lacework of thin black lines going to all of the internal organs. The white coloured nerves that also emerge from the spinal cord go to your muscles and skin sensors.

The Autonomic Nervous System runs automatically – hence its name! Because it is 'automatic', you cannot control it by your thoughts. It works through the unconscious part of your brain. However, your emotions do have a very big influence on this system – it converts your emotions into bodily symptoms and feelings.

The organs that are under the command of the Autonomic Nervous System include:

o   Cardiovascular – your heart and blood vessels
o   Gut – your intestines and bowel
o   Bladder and uterus
o   Glands – your pancreas, gall bladder, sweat glands and saliva glands.

These organs are all connected by the vast nerve network of your 'tummy brain'.

Nerve networks of the tummy brain

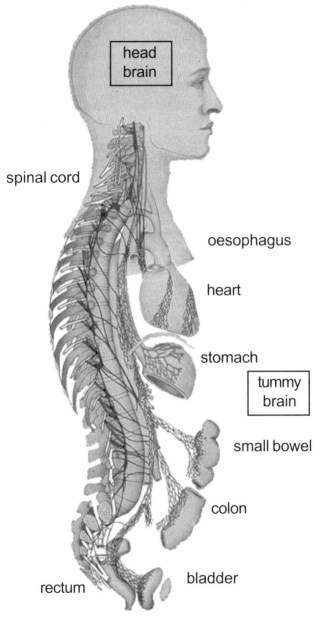

head
brain

spinal cord

oesophagus

heart

stomach

tummy
brain

small bowel

colon

bladder

rectum

The spectrum of neurological symptoms that have been documented as associated with gluten reactions in coeliac disease is as follows:

Neurological conditions associated with gluten

Brain dysfunction
    Headaches and Migraine
    Cerebellar ataxia
    Myoclonic ataxia
    Chronic neuropathies
    Autonomic neuropathy
    Epilepsy
    Dementia

Myopathy

Mood and Behaviour problems
    Anger
    Learning disorders
    Lethargy, low energy
    Attention-deficit/hyperactivity disorder (ADHD)
    Autism
    Depression
    Psychiatric disorders
    Schizophrenia
    Multiple Sclerosis

Gut problems
    Reflux
    Constipation
    Diarrhoea
    Abdominal pain

History of neurological dysfunction and gluten

The first report linking neurological disorders with adult coeliac disease was published over 40 years ago (in 1966) by Cooke and Thomas-Smith. The underlying argument of this and many other similar reports was that gut disease was a prerequisite for these neurological problems, but thirty years later, Marios Hadjivassiliou and others showed that neurological dysfunction could not only precede coeliac disease but could also be its only manifestation (Hadjivassiliou, 1996). Another ten years on and gluten-sensitivity, without histological gut damage, had been clearly shown to cause neurological dysfunction (Hadjivassiliou, 2006).

These links between coeliac disease and brain malfunction have been closely investigated by Zelnik (2004). Patients with coeliac disease were asked to fill out a questionnaire about any neurological problems that they might have had. They were then studied further, and their neurological information was compared with that of a control group.

Zelnik found that coeliac patients were very much more likely to have neurological disorders (51.4%) than the control subjects (19.9%). These neurological disorders included hypotonia, developmental delay, learning disorders and ADHD (attention deficit hyperactivity disorder), headache and cerebella ataxia. Interestingly, epileptic disorders were only marginally more common.

Next, all these subjects were placed on gluten-free diets. A therapeutic benefit of a gluten-free diet was demonstrated in patients with transient infantile hypotonia and migraine headache. Others did not improve. They concluded that their study had shown that the extent of neurological disorders that occurred in people with coeliac disease was much broader than

93

had previously been reported. More than half were affected, however not all of them responded positively to a gluten-free diet. Perhaps if you have a long-standing brain disorder caused by gluten it becomes irreversible with increased time and damage.

Autonomic neuropathy

To recap, your autonomic nervous system takes care of vital day-to-day bodily functions that you never have to think about. This system keeps going day and night. It keeps you breathing, keeps your heart pumping, and keeps your gut working faultlessly. Although it is not under your conscious control, it is strongly influenced by your emotions. Control of your swallowing, your stomach emptying, the flow of food through your intestines and your colonic movements are all mediated through this system.

Usai (1977) also researched this topic carefully. His group investigated the upper-gut motor activity in thirty coeliac patients, looking at the role played by the autonomic nervous system in these motility disturbances.

They also found oesophageal motor abnormalities in half of their patients. Abnormal oesophageal acid studies (pH-probes) were abnormal in 30% of cases and delayed gastric emptying was documented in 50% of the subjects. In total, 75% of coeliac patients were shown to have some sort of gastro-intestinal motility alteration. Tests of autonomic dysfunction were positive in 45% of these patients. This indicated that a gluten autonomic neuropathy was playing a role in their reflux.

Neural antibodies

One mechanism of such nerve damage is through autoimmune damage. A number of nerve and brain antibodies have been detected. For example, one study demonstrated 'anti-ganglioside' antibodies in 64% of patients with coeliac disease who had also been troubled with some sort of neuropathy (Volta, 2006). These auto-antibodies have been shown to bind to a number of critical nerve sites that will go on to damage the nerve. They have been shown to attack the 'Schwann cell' surface, part of the protective coating of the nerve, and also the axons in peripheral nerves.

Gluten-driven brain inflammation

The mechanism by which gluten damages the brain is still uncertain. It might be that IgG-gliadin antibodies interact directly with the nervous system. A patient is described by Ghezzi (in 1997) in a case report which demonstrates a gluten-driven inflammation. This patient had both coeliac disease and progressive brain symptoms (suggesting brain-stem and cerebella involvement), and was subjected to a series of MRI brain scans. The first examination showed multiple brain lesions. Soon after, a large cerebella lesion appeared, and this was followed by severe cerebella atrophy. The presence of structural neuronal damage was confirmed by another type of brain scan (proton MR spectroscopy and magnetization transfer imaging). The MRI results and spinal fluid tests suggested that these neurological complications were more likely to be the result of an inflammatory process.

Evidence of nerve damage

There are some very sensitive cells in the cerebellum (the part of the brain responsible for coordination) called 'Purkinje cells' which function as the output neurons of the cerebellum. These are the cells that appear to be most susceptible to damage by gluten.

Additionally, it has been found that antibodies that attack gluten (the IgG-gliadin antibodies) actually cross-react with these Purkinje cells (Hadjivassiliou, 2002). This means that although an initial immune reaction is mounted against the gluten protein, by chance, this antibody also reacts to the Purkinje nerve cells. This is a 'fatal attraction' which goes on to trigger the subsequent nerve damage in the cerebellum. The outcome is ataxia (poor coordination).

Immune complex disease

Another explanation for the ongoing neuronal malfunction is an inflammatory reaction to gluten in and around the nerve tissues. There is good evidence for this. When gluten gets into the body, it stimulates the production of gluten antibodies by the immune system. The next phase is the formation of 'gluten/gluten-antibody' immune complex reactions. Although this may start off as a non-specific inflammatory reaction, nerve tissue is very sensitive to surrounding inflammatory activity.

Excitotoxins

The activity of excitotoxins is another factor that can invoke neurological damage. Excitotoxins are biochemical substances (usually amino acids) that can react with special neuronal receptors called 'glutamate receptors'. This can happen in both the brain and the spinal cord. This type of reaction is harmful (note that these substances are toxins) and can cause injury to, or even the death of, neurons.

These chemicals are called excitotoxins because they are neurotransmitters (such as glutamate or aspartate) which, in excessive levels, can excite the nerves to death. It is therefore crucial that the levels of these neurotransmitters are properly regulated. If a high level of these neurotransmitters is generated in a normally functioning nerve, they are then re-converted to the more calming neurotransmitter, called GABA, but if a nerve is in an inflamed state, this might not happen. Nerve death occurs when an excess of these excitotoxins causes an imbalance in the flow of calcium into the nerve cell. This leads to the activation of an inflammatory cascade, and the subsequent release of even more inflammatory substances. This leads to neural malfunction and eventual nerve cell death. It is entirely possible that gluten or the 'gluten/antibody immune complex' might act to disturb this delicate balance.

Gastro-intestinal motility disorder

Coeliac patients often show gastro-intestinal motor abnormalities. When asked about 'dyspeptic symptoms', half of all people with coeliac disease say that they have epigastric discomfort (a symptom of heartburn and reflux) or early satiety (feeling full quickly and not wanting to eat any more).

This indicates the presence of a gastro-intestinal motility disorder. This has been further studied by Tursi (2004) who documented disturbed motility of the oesophagus, stomach, small intestine, gallbladder and colon of untreated coeliac patients. The symptoms of the gastro-intestinal malfunction of autonomic motility vary depending on the particular gastro-intestinal zone that is affected. The symptoms that you might experience are:

o   Slow or uncomfortable swallowing (from slower oesophageal transit)

o   Feeling of a full tummy for longer, or inability to eat very much (from delay in the gastric emptying)

o   Nausea or smelly stools (from impaired gallbladder emptying, hence fat digestion problems)

o   Abdominal bloating, gas and tummy pain (from slower orocecal transit time, i.e. food taking a long time to go through your gut)

o   Diarrhoea (from a faster colonic transit time).

These alterations in your gut function are the result of the complex interactions in the gastro-intestinal tract. The results of an impairment of this interweaving of function include the reduced absorption of food nutrients (in particular fat), neurological malfunctions, gut hormonal impairment and small intestinal bacterial overgrowth (from the predisposing motility disorder).

For coeliacs, all these alterations in function should disappear once they go on a gluten-free diet, however the same outcome has also been shown to occur in relation to *The Gluten Syndrome*. All of these gut motility disorders can occur in cases of gluten-sensitivity without the need for additional small bowel histological damage. These symptoms do not stem from tissue damage of the gut – they are caused by neurological damage.

Gastro-oesophageal reflux

Reflux, or heartburn, occurs when the stomach contents are regurgitated back up into the oesophagus. The acid in the stomach causes an irritation, and then a burning of the skin of the oesophagus. This is very uncomfortable. It hurts, and you can experience a burning feeling coming up from your stomach and into your chest. It can even come up into your throat. You can get a really sore chest or a high tummy pain. Babies scream and cry, and toddlers whine, moan and get distressed. Older children experience regurgitation of acid in their mouth and often want to drink milk.

In my experience, both children and adults who have troublesome gastro-oesophageal reflux symptoms are frequently gluten-sensitive. In my studies, I have found that children who have ongoing severe reflux (those who need continued treatment with acid suppressant medication for more than two years) nearly all turn out to be gluten-sensitive. These children have high IgG-gliadin antibody levels. When these children go onto a gluten-free diet, they settle down, they sleep well for the first time and they begin to eat normally. They can usually be weaned off their medications within a few months. Their parents are extremely relieved when they find that their distressing problems have been solved at last.

Gastric reflux is extremely common. Anti-reflux medications are second only to pain killers in terms of numbers prescribed. It is so common that people have come to think that it is a 'normal' symptom. From dealing with these problems every day, I have found that it is usually precipitated by gluten. Most people with gastric reflux have *The Gluten Syndrome.*

Constipation and soiling

When your colon is not functioning properly, you can experience constipation, soiling (encopresis), bloating and, at times, diarrhoea. You can also have a lowered immune function, because your colon is a very important part of your immune system.

To empty out your colon, your large bowel muscles have to work efficiently to move the faecal contents along. You also have to be able to feel the 'call to stool' – that is, the urge to download. I have found that children (and adults) with constipation as a result of gluten-sensitivity have poor sensations about wanting to defecate. They cannot feel it coming. This is due to damage to the nerves that control this function. Once they go gluten-free, it usually takes about 3–6 months for everything to come right again.

Much more evidence

There are numerous other symptoms that provide evidence that problems are stemming from dysfunction of the Autonomic Nervous System caused by gluten. This is fully documented in my book *Full of it! The shocking truth about gluten.*

An underlying nutritional deficiency alone cannot explain these neuromuscular disorders. There are a number of arguments in support of this:

o   Many of the neuromuscular disorders that are described in association with coeliac disease and gluten-sensitivity have an inflammatory or autoimmune basis which cannot be generated simply by food deficiencies
o   Many neurological disorders are seen in the complete absence of any gastro-intestinal disorder
o   Many people with gluten-related neuropathy have no physical or biochemical evidence of malabsorption or nutritional deficiency.

Gluten the troublemaker

There is abundant evidence that gluten is the troublemaker in the brain. Therefore, there is no need to invoke coeliac disease as the culprit. The overall condition is called *The Gluten Syndrome*. To conclude:

1) A brain disease

I believe that gluten-sensitivity is primarily a neurological problem. A major contributing factor to this debate has been the realization that the brain has a central role in the expression of the symptoms that have until now been attributed to the local toxicity of gluten on the gut. Traditionally, gluten reactions have been thought to be a result of gluten directly damaging the gut tissue. However, all of these symptoms can now be explained through their brain connections and the subsequent disorder of their feedback mechanisms.

2) A nerve disease

I propose that gluten-sensitivity is also a nerve disease. There is a gigantic network of nerves that controls every function that your gut is programmed to perform. There are as many nerve cells in your gut as there are in your head – about 25 billion! I call it your 'tummy brain' (or 'gut brain'). Your tummy brain can be directly damaged by gluten reactions. This is the cause of so many sore tummies and bowel problems.

3) A wide spectrum of neurological manifestations

For decades there have been reports of unexplained brain and nerve symptoms associated with coeliac disease. Although these associations have been noted and described, no universal mechanism has been proposed. However, if gluten is regarded as a neurotoxin, then the explanation has been found. This toxicity may act through inflammatory mechanisms.

4) A very common disease

Reactions to gluten have been documented as being extremely common. About one in ten people (as ascertained by blood donor studies) have high levels of gluten antibodies in their blood. My clinical studies have confirmed this number of gluten-sensitive people. Many population studies on coeliac disease have found that about one in every hundred people are affected, therefore I have demonstrated that coeliac disease comprises only one-tenth of the gluten problem.

Are you affected?

This 'brain and nerves' theory underlying *The Gluten Syndrome* is attractive because it provides a unifying solution to the conundrums associated with gluten. It explains: the mechanism of the non-gut symptoms of coeliac disease; the behaviour disturbance side of gluten reactions; the psychiatric and personality disorders; the neurological symptoms; the autonomic system disturbances; and why such small amounts of gluten can cause such major reactions (by the amplification effect of the nervous system).

The shocking truth about gluten is that it can damage your brain and nerves. People are encouraged to eat gluten foods, but this might be steadily eroding their health and energy. If you have any lingering doubts about your own health, I suggest you check out the possibility that you might have *The Gluten Syndrome*.

The Gluten Syndrome – are you affected?

6. Glutened patients

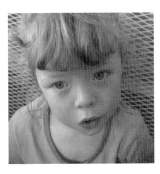

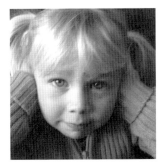

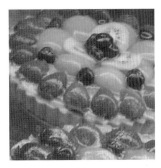

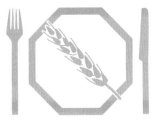

6. Glutened patients

Many people who experience an unpleasant reaction to gluten say that they have been 'glutened'. Over the last ten years I have diagnosed and helped thousands of patients whose symptoms have been associated with eating gluten. These people have *The Gluten Syndrome*. I have listened to their troubles, which had often previously been played down by some other practitioners.

These patients and parents often felt that the medical fraternity had turned a deaf ear to their condition. The children were sometimes labelled as 'naughty' and the parents had often been blamed for their child's symptoms.

In previous chapters I have outlined my ideas and presented supporting evidence from the literature for the diagnosis of *The Gluten Syndrome*. I now present you with a clinical audit of nearly a thousand children and their families, and ask that you draw your own conclusions.

This analysis shows that *The Gluten Syndrome*:
o   is an important and common condition
o   affects about one in ten people
o   can be readily identified by the IgG-gliadin blood test
o   responds dramatically to a gluten-free diet
o   includes gluten-sensitive people both with and without gut damage (i.e. coeliac disease).

Background

To put this clinical survey into context, I first want to emphasize some of the elements that place my arguments apart from many others. I am looking at: 1) the symptoms, not just the gut tissue; 2) the gluten antibodies, not just the tissue antibodies; and 3) the brain, not just the gut. Let's examine these three key points in more detail.

1. Look at the symptoms, not just the gut tissue

My fundamental principle is that the primary symptoms of gluten-sensitivity arise from *gluten reactivity* rather than as a result of gut damage. Therefore, this audit is directed towards my patients' symptoms rather than a tissue-based diagnosis of coeliac disease. However, in order to satisfy those of my colleagues who are gut-biopsy orientated, I have also carried out an analysis of biopsy-only subjects.

In the context of this analysis, coeliac disease is defined as a tissue diagnosis (rather than a clinical diagnosis): the term coeliac disease is confined to those people who have been investigated and shown to have an abnormal small bowel biopsy. This gut damage, which is caused by gluten, only appears in genetically-susceptible people. It is detected by looking at a piece of tissue under a microscope (this is called histology). This tissue is obtained by a procedure called an upper gastrointestinal endoscopy.

Symptoms are important

-----

2. Look at the gluten antibodies, not just the tissue antibodies

To date, in the medical world, the development of blood tests has focused almost exclusively on making an accurate diagnosis of coeliac disease. In order to do this, any blood test results have had to be compared with evidence of tissue damage.

Two categories of blood test have been developed: one, the gluten test (IgG-gliadin), detects antibodies to gliadin (or gluten). The other, the tissue damage test (tTG), detects antibodies to damaged small bowel tissue (see Chapter 2 for more detail).

In short, these two tests measure two very different things. In coeliac disease, both tests are usually positive. If you were to be only interested in coeliac disease, then any potential test that was not consistently found to be associated with tissue damage would be declared 'non-specific'. Under this premise, the gluten antibody (IgG-gliadin) test is a poor predictor of coeliac disease: it is 'non-specific' for coeliac disease.

By contrast, the tissue antibody (tTG) test is an excellent predictor of coeliac disease. Consequently, the medical profession is gradually discarding the IgG-gliadin test, however this is a case of throwing the baby out with the bath water. In my clinical practice I have found that the IgG-gliadin test is an excellent predictor of *The Gluten Syndrome*.

IgG-gliadin antibodies indicate a reaction to gluten

Gluten antibodies. Your immune system is always on the lookout for foreign proteins that are constantly invading your body. Gluten is one such protein. Evidence of this immune reaction is provided by the production of the 'IgG-anti-gliadin antibody' (often shortened to 'IgG-gliadin'). The IgG-gliadin test does not reliably identify people with coeliac disease (those with tissue damage), but it does detect people who are gluten-sensitive. Currently, this is the aspect of gluten intolerance that has been ignored by the medical community. The purpose of this audit is to present data supporting the entity of *The Gluten Syndrome*.

3. Look at the brain, not just at the gut

Your 'tummy brain' refers to the vast networks of nerves, cells and fibres that lace your gastrointestinal tract. These nerves link your brain directly to your gut. Your thoughts and emotions also directly affect your gut through this nerve network. Conversely, your gut can affect your brain.

Eating should be both pleasurable and comfortable for you. If it is not, then something is wrong. Now there is evidence that gluten can damage your brain and nerves. This 'brain symptom' evidence from brain-imaging and brain-cell research is overwhelming. The evidence places the damage by gluten squarely in the neural tissues.

Clinical observations of gluten patients

Let me introduce you to nearly one thousand children. This is a clinical survey of my patients, who were seen in my gastroenterology and allergy clinic in Christchurch, New Zealand. Information was extracted retrospectively for the six years from 2001 to 2006.

The purpose of this survey was to determine the number of children who were sensitive to gluten in their diet. The majority of these patients did not have coeliac disease. I also wanted to document the value of the IgG-gliadin blood test for the diagnosis of gluten-sensitivity.

Blood tests. Blood tests were requested for all patients who had: chronic gut symptoms; suspicion of having coeliac disease; chronic eczema; poor health; poor growth; possible nutritional deficiency; or immunological problems. Many patients had two or more blood tests during the survey period.

The blood tests that are reported are: IgG-gliadin; IgA-gliadin; tissue transglutaminase (tTG); and endomesial antibodies (EMA).

Endoscopy tests: If warranted, an endoscopy was organized in order to obtain a small bowel biopsy, and also to look at the oesophagus and stomach. These biopsy findings were analysed in relation to the patients' symptoms and blood tests.

Analysis and results

The focus of this patient survey was to examine the clinical value of the IgG-gliadin test, however there was a primary interest in who might have coeliac disease. This was due to current medical teaching which states that the only condition gluten can cause is coeliac disease. Therefore, the data is presented as follows:

1) You are shown the profile of the children that I investigated

2) The small bowel biopsy data are presented. There were 217 children who were investigated by endoscopy to determine if they had histological coeliac disease. The coeliac children were then compared to the rest of the biopsy group.

3) Information on the 724 children who had raised IgG-gliadin antibody levels is presented.

1) The children

There were 921 children (aged 18 years and younger) included in this survey who all met the following criteria:

o   Had blood tests for both IgG-gliadin and tTG (or EMA)
o   Had the last blood test within the previous five years
o   Had been eating gluten prior to their first blood test
o   Had at least three months of clinical follow-up
     information available.

These children had an average age of 5.3 years (ranging from 4 months to 18 years) and there was an even gender distribution: 493 males and 428 females.

Their symptoms are listed in the table in order of frequency of occurrence. In total, 596 children (67%) had some sort of gut symptoms, and nearly half had experienced abdominal pain.

Symptoms of 921 children investigated for possible gluten reactions

Gut symptoms 67%

Abdominal pain	42%
Diarrhoea	23%
Constipation	13%
Vomiting	7%
Gastric reflux	24%

Growth concerns 40%

Poor weight	24%
Poor height	18%
Pot tummy	17%

Behaviour concerns 49%

Irritable	27%
Hyperactive/defiant	8%
Poor sleep	12%
Tired/lethargic	22%
Headache	9%
Delayed development	3%

Allergy/Immune issues 52%

Eczema	32%
CMA/Food allergy	29%
Run down	16%

N.B.: The total percentage of patients in each category does not equal the sum of those exhibiting the symptoms described because most of these children had a combination of problems.

This list of symptoms is illustrative of the range of children that are brought to me for investigation of their problems. I am a paediatric gastroenterologist and allergist, and their symptoms reflect this speciality. I have divided their symptoms into four categories: gut symptoms; growth concerns; behaviour concerns; and allergy/immune issues.

All of these children were investigated with blood tests. There were 724 (79%) with high IgG-gliadin levels (>14 units). There were 217 children who were investigated by endoscopy. Those with blood tests that supported the diagnosis of *The Gluten Syndrome* were offered a trial with a gluten-free diet.

2) The 217 biopsy children

Endoscopy

The endoscopy procedure is a crucial investigation to determine if and where there is small bowel tissue damage.

The term 'villous atrophy' is used to describe the classical biopsy changes seen in coeliac disease. As the current diagnosis of coeliac disease is based on the appearance of the small bowel tissue, it cannot be diagnosed in the absence of small bowel damage (although biopsy results are not always reliable – see Chapter 2).

To summarise, the endoscopic biopsy is troubled by a number of factors: the damage can be patchy and therefore be missed; the damage may be very subtle, and therefore missed by an inexperienced histologist; the damage can sometimes only be seen by an electron microscope; or the child might not yet have any damage because not enough gluten has been ingested.

Consequently, the biopsy cannot be seen as the 'gold standard'. It is able to confirm coeliac disease – but it cannot rule it out.

Nevertheless, additional important information can be gained from endoscopy. Samples of tissue can also be taken from the oesophagus and from the stomach. In addition, the function of the small bowel can be assessed by measuring the enzyme activity of the disaccharidases (lactase, maltase and sucrase) in small bowel tissue. The guidelines that I use to determine who should have a small bowel biopsy are:

o   Elevated tTG or EMA antibodies
o   Elevated IgA-gliadin levels (usually IgG-gliadin is also substantially raised)
o   High IgG-gliadin levels with symptoms despite no family history
o   Those who are failing to thrive (poor growth) without explanation and who have negative coeliac and gluten antibody markers
o   Persistent clinical gastro-oesophageal reflux.

In my experience, the small bowel biopsy is usually histologically normal in children over five years of age who have minor symptoms and who have only moderately elevated IgG-gliadin, with normal tTG levels.

Biopsy results

There were 217 children (24% of the total sample of 921 children) who had a small bowel biopsy. Their average age was 5.5 years (standard deviation 3.9 years).

The biopsy findings of these 217 children were:
o   31 had coeliac histology
o   45 had evidence of oesophagitis
o   81 had low disaccharidases enzymes
o   95 displayed no abnormalities using these conventional means.

In total, abnormalities were found in 122 (56%) of these biopsies, with many children displaying several abnormalities in their results. To make sense of this information, the results were placed in mutually exclusive categories and then ranked in order of importance. The highest ranking group was of course the coeliac children (14%); next were those with low disaccharidase enzymes (30%); the third group were those who had oesophagitis only (12%); which left those whose endoscopies showed no abnormalities (44%) in the final group. These findings are listed in the table below:

Ranking of biopsy results

Biopsy result	Number (n=217)
Coeliac histology	31 (14%) (16 also had low enzymes and 3 had oesophagitis)
Low enzymes	65 (30%) (16 also had oesophagitis)
Oesophagitis only	26 (12%)
Normal	95 (44%)

This grouping of biopsy results was then used to look at the blood test results for both gluten and tissue antibody tests.

Biopsy results compared with ttG blood tests

This graph shows the relationship between the biopsy findings and the tTG (tissue transglutaminase) blood test levels. On the x-axis are the four categories of the biopsy result. The y-axis shows the tTG levels (normal being less than 20 units, shown by the dashed line).

Comparison between tTG levels by small bowel biopsy result (n=217)

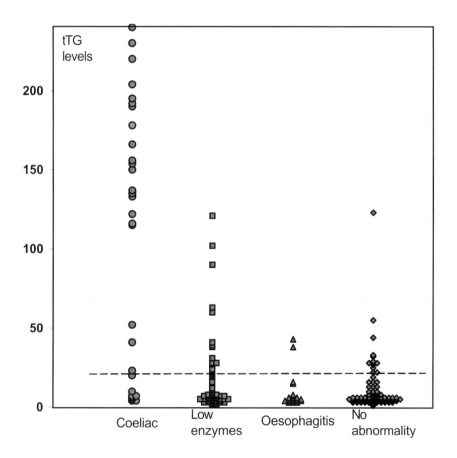

High tTG levels. Clearly, the coeliac group had the highest tTG levels. This indicates that if the tTG is over 100 units, then histological confirmation of coeliac disease is almost a certainty. However most whose tTG levels were between 20–100 did not have coeliac disease.

Low tTG and coeliac disease. It is of interest that there are 8 coeliac children with 'normal' levels of tTG. The details of their results are shown in the table below, in order of age. The cut-off for normal antibody levels is shown in brackets. A level higher than this is abnormal.

Details of 8 coeliac children with 'normal' levels of tTG

Child	Age (yr-mo)	tTG (>20)	IgG-gliadin (>20)	IgA-gliadin (>15)	IgA Deficiency
1	0–10	20	45	2	no
2	0–11	4	18	5	no
3	1–4	10	156	49	no
4	1–7	5	75	40	no
5	3–1	6	100	10	no
6	4–6	4	65	8	no
7	8–10	7	66	11	yes
8	11–3	7	126	15	no

The important observations to make from this table are:
o   Only one of these 8 children had IgA-deficiency
o   Their ages ranged from 10 months through to 11 years, but only two were over the age of five
o   Three had high IgA-gliadin levels, often a good indicator of intestinal damage
o   Most (7 of the 8) had substantially raised IgG-gliadin levels.

ttG not so accurate

The main conclusion to be drawn from this information is that the ttG antibody test is not accurate enough to be able to be relied on to make a diagnosis of coeliac disease in all children (Trevisiol et al., 2002).

Additionally, the IgG-gliadin and IgA-gliadin antibody tests are valuable ancillary tests that can be used to reveal the existence of coeliac disease in children.

High ttG and low enzymes. The next important point to ponder is that high ttG levels were found in 15 (23%) of the 65 children in the low enzyme group (those with depressed activity of their dissacharidase enzymes in the small bowel tissue).

One interpretation of this finding is that these children are developing gut damage, which is not yet severe enough to show up under a microscope. There is good evidence for this idea. If a very high-powered microscope is used (an electron microscope), then abnormalities of the gut can be found in about half of such children (Sarbati et al., 2003).

The meaning of a high ttG. The last point that I wish to make from the study of the ttG data is that of the 57 children with a high ttG level, less than half (23 children or 40%) were confirmed to have coeliac disease by their biopsy histology. So, what does the raised ttG level mean in these children without the coeliac histology? It is my experience that most of these children also have a high IgG-gliadin antibody level, and their symptoms improve on a gluten-free diet.

It is also my experience that the majority of these children will eventually develop the full picture of coeliac disease if they are left on gluten. The small bowel damage can occur gradually. This means that in the early stages of coeliac disease there is no visible small bowel damage. Such thinking therefore makes nonsense of the mandate that histological damage must be present before coeliac disease can be diagnosed! Surely a revision of the criteria for the diagnosis of coeliac disease, without the need for villous atrophy to be in evidence, is called for.

If the tTG level is up, but the histology is normal, it could mean that this person might eventually develop coeliac disease.

I now put these patients on a gluten-free diet, and their symptoms invariably remit. Clearly, the small bowel biopsy is not the last word in diagnosis.

A gluten-free diet should not hinge on the biopsy result

Biopsy results compared with IgG-gliadin tests

Next we will look at the IgG-gliadin antibody levels in relation to the small bowel histology appearances. Again, the x-axis on the graph shows the four categories of biopsy result. The y-axis indicates the IgG-gliadin levels (normal being less than 20 units, shown by the dashed line).

Comparison between IgG-gliadin levels by small bowel biopsy result (n=217)

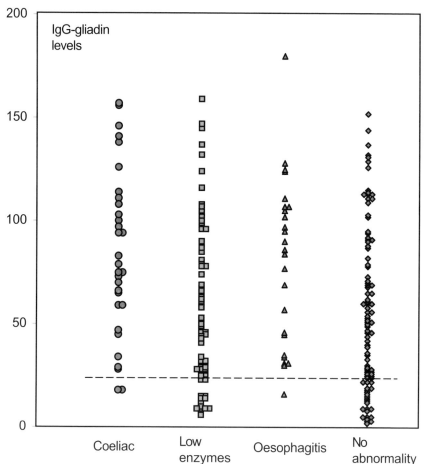

From the graph you can easily see that it is impossible to distinguish between the four groups on the basis of the IgG-gliadin level.

One of the prerequisite criteria necessary for an endoscopy was a high IgG-gliadin level, something that needs to be borne in mind when interpreting these results. Setting the cut-off value for IgG-gliadin is not a straight-forward exercise. The laboratory states that a level of 20 units or greater is abnormal, however in my experience a lower cut-off level of about 15 is more applicable to children (this cut-off will be used in the next section). Nevertheless, the 20 unit cut-off level is used for this analysis.

The points to take from this graph showing the results of these 217 children are:

o   84% (182 of 217) of these children had high IgG-gliadin levels
o   94% (29 of 31) in the coeliac group had high IgG-gliadin levels
o   The averages and ranges of the IgG-gliadin results were similar in all four groups
o   The IgG-gliadin result was not predictive of abnormal small bowel histology.

Coeliac 'categories'

The primary role of an endoscopy (also called a small bowel biopsy) is to establish whether or not there is any tissue damage. However, as stated above, it is an imperfect test. So, in order to be as clear cut as possible, I have established three coeliac 'categories' based on a combination of histology and blood test results.

o   *Definite* coeliac disease: those with definite coeliac histology on biopsy regardless of the blood test results (n = 31)

o   *Possible* coeliac disease: those with an elevation of their tissue antibody tests (tTG and/or EMA) but with normal gut histology. This is the half-way group. These children could possibly go on to develop established histological disease if they were left on gluten for a much longer time (n = 38)

o   *Not* coeliac disease: those with both an apparently 'normal' small bowel and 'normal' levels of tissue antibodies. The term 'normal' is shown in quote marks because the establishment of normal values is problematical, however at the time of endoscopy they did not show any histological evidence of small bowel damage (n = 148).

Symptoms seen in the coeliac 'categories'

A startling finding was that there were no distinguishing symptoms that could explicitly identify coeliac disease. In other words, the 31 children who had the gut tissue damage of coeliac disease could not be singled out from the others on the basis of their symptoms alone.

The symptoms experienced by these 217 children, placed in their coeliac categories, are presented in the table below. There was no sure-fire way to distinguish these three groups by their symptoms alone. Symptoms were grouped into gut symptoms, behaviour concerns, growth concerns, and allergy/immune problems.

The coeliac group had fewer food allergies and slightly higher numbers of pot tummies, however it is clear that the only way to detect coeliac disease is through a combination of blood tests and endoscopy.

Coeliacs cannot be distinguished by their symptoms

Symptoms experienced by the 217 children who had biopsies, placed in their coeliac categories

	Definite coeliac (n=31)	*Possible* coeliac (n=38)	*Not* coeliac (n=148)
Gut symptoms	**87%**	**79%**	**82%**
Abdominal pain	48%	50%	50%
Diarrhoea	45%	34%	32%
Constipation	6%	26%	12%
Vomiting	6%	11%	13%
Gastric reflux	16%	18%	30%
Behaviour concerns	**71%**	**50%**	**50%**
Tired/lethargic	48%	34%	23%
Irritable	35%	45%	34%
Poor sleep	16%	13%	15%
Headache	16%	11%	9%
Delayed development	3%	3%	2%
Hyperactive/defiant	10%	11%	7%
Growth concerns	**61%**	**53%**	**52%**
Poor weight	32%	29%	37%
Poor height	35%	32%	29%
Pot tummy	29%	24%	20%
Allergy/Immune issues	**39%**	**39%**	**46%**
Eczema	26%	21%	29%
CMA/Food allergy	13%	18%	24%
Run down	16%	18%	18%

Who warrants a gluten-free diet?

Conventionally, only confirmed coeliacs are put on a gluten-free diet, but the big question that few people have asked before is: "Do children with high levels of gluten antibodies, but without evidence of coeliac disease, respond to a gluten-free diet?"

Who should go onto a gluten-free diet? Finding an answer to this question was the central purpose of this study. My main interest was in observing how the group of *'Not* coeliac' children would respond to a gluten-free diet.

The answer is presented in the table below in the form of a comparison between the three groups who went gluten-free and their subsequent outcomes. Subjects were deemed to have improved if their parents reported that they were better on the gluten-free diet (and usually also reported that when they accidentally ingested gluten their symptoms returned).

Gluten-free diet outcome by coeliac category

	Definite coeliac (n=31)	*Possible* coeliac (n=38)	*Not* coeliac (n=148)
ImprovedGluten-free			
Calculated by those who **tried a gluten-free diet**	29/31 (94%)	27/38 (71%)	93/102 (91%)

It is not surprising that 94% of the *'Definite* coeliacs' improved, in fact the only two who did not improve had no symptoms to start with and were picked up by family testing!

A positive response was also seen in the *'Possible* coeliac' group, with 71% improving when off gluten. This is an interesting result. Perhaps these children had early coeliac disease: too early to detect by histology, but showing early signs of tissue damage nevertheless.

In summary, of the '*Not* coeliac' group, there were 44 who did not try a gluten-free diet, and of the 102 who did, only 11 showed no improvement. This is a remarkable finding. These children were sensitive to gluten, but showed no evidence of coeliac disease. They are indicative of *The Gluten Syndrome.*

Intention to treat: Clinical audits can be complicated by unreliability of subjects: sometimes it wasn't possible to collect all the necessary information from follow up visits; sometimes people did not follow the advice given; and sometimes children were already on a diet that excluded other food groups such as dairy and egg, therefore it was inappropriate for them to trial a gluten-free diet.

Because of these limitations, I have also analysed the numbers in the harshest way possible: this is called 'intention to treat'. This means that in cases where there was inadequate information, these children were deemed not to have improved. This approach underestimates any benefits achieved by a gluten-free diet.

'Intention to treat' outcome of a gluten-free diet by coeliac category

	Definite coeliac (n=31)	Possible coeliac (n=38)	Not coeliac (n=148)
ImprovedGluten-free			
Calculated by **intention to treat**	29/31 (94%)	27/38 (71%)	93/148 (63%)

Of the '*Not* coeliac' group, 63% (93 of 148) reported substantial clinical improvements on a gluten-free diet. Of the other 55 children, there were 44 who did not try a gluten-free diet (usually owing to other food restriction at the time of assessment), and 11 reported no benefit. So, even using the most stringent means of analysis, over half of the *'Not* coeliac' group improved substantially on a gluten-free diet.

Who improved when going gluten-free?

So, which children were most likely to improve on a gluten-free diet? To answer this question, I have once again compared the three groups. Interestingly, there were no real differences in terms of gender or average age. The age of discovery of the coeliac children (average age of 6.0 years) was dependent on their age of referral to me. Some had been ill for longer than others.

Characteristics of children who improved on a gluten-free diet

	Definite coeliac (n=29)	*Possible* coeliac (n=27)	*Not* coeliac (n=93)
Gender			
Girls	43%	27%	54%
Boys	57%	73%	46%
Age in years			
Average age	6.0	6.4	5.0
Standard deviation	4.2	3.3	3.8

I had expected to find that the '*Possible* coeliacs' were younger on average than the '*Definite* coeliacs', but that turned out not to be the case.

125

Negative gliadin antibodies but a gluten-free response

Based on my clinical experience, I am strongly influenced by the IgG-gliadin antibody levels when deciding to recommend a gluten-free diet. However, over the years I have placed seven children (who were not included in this study) on a gluten-free diet despite their test results indicating 'normal' antibody levels.

In each instance, this was because other members in the household were already on a gluten-free diet, and the child was displaying symptoms of gluten-sensitivity. And in each instance, after a short time on a gluten-free diet, their symptoms resolved! This means that a negative result for IgG-gliadin does not necessarily rule out a positive response to a gluten-free diet.

The IgG-gliadin test does not rule out gluten-sensitivity

HLA status

The HLA test only became available part-way through the six year period during which this study was conducted, therefore not all children underwent this test. The HLA test provides information about the genetic possibility of developing the gut damage of coeliac disease. Population studies suggest that between one quarter and one third (25–35%) of the population have the DQ2 and/or the DQ8 HLA gene. About 95% of coeliacs are positive to one or both of these HLA types.

In this clinical study, a total of 67 children were tested, of whom 48 (72%) proved positive. The breakdown by group is shown in the table below. A high incidence of these genes was seen in all three groups, suggesting that *The Gluten Syndrome* is, in some way, genetically predisposed.

HLA status of children who improved on a gluten-free diet

	Definite coeliac (n=16)	*Possible* coeliac (n=13)	*Not* coeliac (n=38)
HLA Gene tests			
HLA positive for DQ2 and/or DQ	14 (88%)	9 (69%)	25 (66%)

(A total of 67 children were tested, of whom 48 (72%) proved positive)

The Gluten Syndrome runs in families

127

What the parents said

I have already outlined the types of symptoms that these children were experiencing, but the following statements are from verbatim accounts provided by the parents and children after the children had spent three months on a gluten-free diet. They were asked to comment on how they felt they were progressing. This is what they said:

Comments from '*Not* coeliac' group and their parents after experiencing a gluten-free diet for three months

Really good gluten-free, growing very well.

Still some sore tummies.

Better! Used to blink all the time but now okay, eczema gone.

All his symptoms have disappeared, gets sore tummy with gluten.

No symptoms now, better at school, concentration better, eating more.

Really good, now eating, bowels normal.

He was able to get off Omeprazole, sleeping good, bowels good, eating well.

Better appetite, able to come off reflux medication.

A different child! No longer tired, not as hypersensitive, bowels normal, tummy good.

Very much better.

Dramatic response, happy again.

Very sensitive to gluten.

Improving and growing, reflux now gone.

Generally better off gluten.

Very sensitive to gluten, gets a bad tummy.

Much better! Bowel motions now better.

Very much better. A completely different girl, happy, settled, eating well.

A different girl.

Gluten-free associated with excellent health.

Took a year to get better.
Growth much improved.
A lot better off gluten.
Very good response initially, reflux gone and felt great.
Immediate improvement. Happier and more settled.
Within a few days a different kid. Happier, more energy, eczema
   cleared.
I feel better. More energy.
Great health on gluten-free.
A lot better gluten-free.
Wow! What a difference, within a week better.
Behaviour change for the better.
No more sore tummies or headaches.
Some improvement.
Better for a few weeks, then relapsed.
Growing again, good health.
Alopecia improving.
Upset by gluten in breast milk.
No more tummy pains or headaches.
Bowel motions normal now, face rash gone, eating better, still not
   sleeping.
Happy on the gluten-free diet, improving.
Tummy better off gluten, mood still diabolical.
Huge difference since gluten-free. Better behaviour, sleeping
   better, happier.
Since gluten-free, growing again, bowels normal and improved
   moods.
Dizzy, runny nose, withdrawn behaviour: all better off gluten.
Improving fast, big difference.
Much better, improved behaviour.
Doing very well.
A lot better, not been sick, more energy, appetite come back.
Head fine, all symptoms okay.
A huge difference. Very very well gluten-free.
Happier, eating better, bowels normal.

Much better, less irritable.

Had poor growth, now more energetic.

Really good since went gluten-free, happy, eating better.

A new child, perked up and thriving.

Improved significantly.

Bloating gone and more energy. Then relapsed with sore tummy and reflux.

Pleased with progress.

Yes, good, better. No tummy or headaches, concentration better.

Asking for food for the first time. No pain!

Made a huge difference, it is miraculous. First time she had had normal bowels.

A different kid, happy, growing again.

Within weeks her eczema went, bowels normal, much more energy.

Really enjoying the diet and feels so much better.

She was able to come off Ritalin, eating so much better.

Improved remarkably well.

Was really good off gluten. But can't stick to the diet.

Tummy pain went immediately. Very great improvement. No more aches and pains.

Moods better, calmer.

After ten days gluten-free his eczema went entirely.

Better!

Really good, no more sore tummies.

Happy, stopped screaming, now can walk and talk.

More energy, tummy okay now, tummy gone down.

Made a huge improvement.

Picked up well, great health.

A lot more energy, tummy good, I feel so much better.

Gluten infringements make him grumpy.

Great! The answer to his health, diarrhoea gone, has got energy.

Eating well and putting on weight.

Tummy pains gone, eczema a bit better.

Excellent. Very sensitive to gluten.

Excellent on gluten-free, growing.
Wonderful, a miracle, lots of energy and bowels normal.
Great! Much better, normal bowels.
Improved considerably, much better.
Upset by small amounts of gluten with pain and distress.
More energetic, happier, more social.
I feel greater than ever, but was very reluctant to go gluten-free.
Much better now, gluten gives him a stomach ache.
More energy, more bounce and tummy good.
Good! Happier, back to normal, happy at last.
No more sore tummies, stopped the reflux, eating better.
A major change in his behaviour, a different boy, able to stop
    Omeprazole.
Put on weight again, but took a long time to get better.
Gluten slip-ups cause sore tummy, headaches, emotional outbursts.
Never gets tummy aches now, but still on Omeprazole.
A radical change! A lot more settled, more focused, more relaxed.
Fuzzy head has gone, more energy.
Very much better off gluten. Also on Omeprazole.
Really good! A different girl.

These statements from the parents and the children themselves
are exciting to read. Many of these children had been unwell
for years. They had tried all sorts of treatments, but it was only
the gluten-free diet that helped them, and if they made gluten
errors, they would experience the return of their symptoms.

These children were prepared to stay strictly gluten-free so that
they could feel well again. Most were highly compliant and
cooperative regarding the diet. Being gluten-free was not much
of a burden to them.

Conclusions

Many children have symptoms consistent with coeliac disease, but have normal small bowel histology and normal tTG or EMA results. However, they frequently have high IgG-gliadin antibody levels.

The results of the study are emphatic – these children also respond to a gluten-free diet, because they are gluten-sensitive. The IgG-gliadin test is crucial in detecting these children. It is clear then that many more children, other than coeliacs, warrant a gluten-free diet.

Many more than coeliacs warrant a gluten-free diet

3) *644 children with high IgG-gliadin levels*

Finally, I would like to tell you a little bit more about the gluten-free outcomes of a larger group of children. These are the 644 children with high IgG-gliadin levels who did not have any evidence of coeliac disease.

To recap, I carried out a survey of 921 children who were referred to my clinic during the period 2001–2006. These children had been investigated for coeliac disease through IgG-gliadin antibody (*Inova Diagnostics*) and tissue transglutaminase (tTG) or endomesial antibody (EMA) blood tests.

There were 723 children with elevated IgG-gliadin levels (>14 units: please note that I have used a slightly lower cut-off point which I have recognised as being of greater clinical relevance for these children). Their average age was 5.3 years (standard deviation 3.8 years). All were offered a gluten-free diet.

They were then placed into the three categories that you are by now familiar with:

o   31 (4.3%) were '*Definite* coeliac' with positive histology diagnosis.

o   48 (6.6%) were deemed '*Possible* coeliac' because despite elevated levels of tTG or EMA antibodies they had a normal small bowel histology.

o   644 (89.1%), who had no evidence of gut damage and no evidence of elevated tissue damage antibodies were labelled '*Not* coeliac'.

Clinical features were similar across these three groups, although the '*Definite* coeliac' group displayed more gut symptoms and fewer food allergies.

The IgG-gliadin antibody levels

The graph shows the IgG-gliadin antibody levels for the 723 children with elevated IgG-gliadin levels (>14 units). As you can see, there is a significant variation in the levels, however as previously noted, a high IgG-gliadin level does not necessarily provide any indication as to the likelihood of tissue damage.

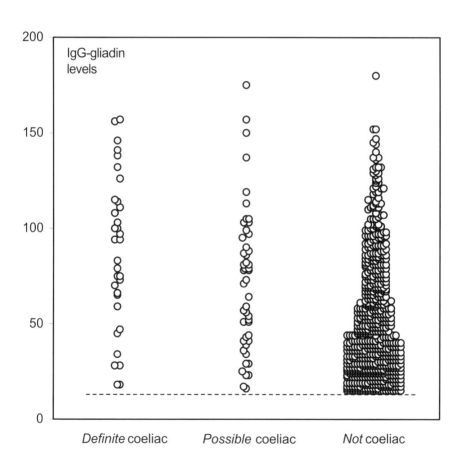

A high level of IgG-gliadin antibody is, however, clearly associated with an improvement in symptoms following time spent on a gluten-free diet: it is, therefore, highly indicative of gluten-sensitivity.

Gluten-free outcomes

The full results are presented in the table below. Of the 644 '*Not* coeliac', all of whom had elevated IgG-gliadin antibody levels, 434 were trialled on a gluten-free diet. A large proportion (343 or 79%) of these children reported a substantial clinical improvement. Either the parent or child said that they were much better.

(When this is calculated on the 'intention to treat' basis, the proportion who showed improvement was seen to be 53%. This lower figure is due to the many patients who did not trial a gluten-free diet for reasons that have been outlined earlier).

Proportion of children who improved on a gluten-free diet

	Improved on gluten-free diet	
	By those who trialled a gluten-free diet	By intention to treat
Patient groups		
Definite coeliac	**29/31 (94%)**	29/31 (94%)
Possible coeliac	**36/48 (75%)**	36/48 (75%)
Not coeliac	**343/434 (79%)**	343/644 (53%)

In the other two groups, improvement was seen in 29 of the 31 '*Definite* coeliac' (94%) and 36 of the 48 '*Possible* coeliac' (75%).

Not coeliacs respond well to a gluten-free diet

What critics say

The medical profession is conservative. It demands a high standard of proof before changing clinical guidelines. But how much proof, and what sort of proof is necessary?

I have already given you the background to the entrenched position on coeliac disease. To recap, the currently held medical view is that coeliac disease is a gut disease and that the only role for a gluten-free diet is for the treatment of a person with the biopsy-proven histological damage of coeliac disease. This book reveals a wider perspective on gluten-sensitivity and I have presented my evidence for this. It is easy to be critical. It is more comfortable to oppose change. It requires courage to put forward a whole new way of thinking about gluten.

Professor Tim Ball, University Winnipeg, Canada, writes about this concept of the acceptance of new ideas: "Until you have challenged the prevailing wisdom you have no idea how nasty people can be. Until you have re-examined any issue in an attempt to find out all the information, you cannot know how much misinformation exists in the supposed age of information."

Criticisms about *The Gluten Syndrome*

I have promoted the concept of gluten-sensitivity and *The Gluten Syndrome* for many years. I have had the opportunity to present this data to a number of international medical conferences. A great number of medical people have told me that they see many of the type of patients that I have described. However, there are also medical critics. Here are some of their criticisms and my responses.

The benefits that your patients experience are subjective

Yes, their reports of the benefits of a gluten-free diet are subjective. In the opinion of the patient, or parent, or child, they say that they feel better and are grateful that their symptoms have disappeared. These families are willing to persevere on a strict gluten-free diet for years because of the benefits that they ascribe to the diet. They find that even small infringements cause a relapse. They report how they feel on a gluten-free diet – this is subjective. These critics readily believe the subjective reports of a "confirmed coeliac" who gets better on a gluten-free diet. So, why do not these same critics accept the similar subjective reports just because the endoscopy does not show any small bowel damage?

The benefits are due to my observation bias

Yes, I am biased. I see many people who react badly to gluten, despite not having coeliac disease. However, I endeavour to be unbiased in my clinical assessment. This bias would be an important factor if my results were borderline. However, I am overwhelmed by the numbers of children and adults who have made dramatic recoveries on a gluten-free diet. Previously, they had experienced ill health for years, or even decades.

The benefits are due to a healthier diet

Yes, a healthier diet will contribute to better health. I emphasize to my patients the need to ensure that iron deficiency and other mineral/vitamin deficits are restored. Iron repletion makes a big difference. However, gluten-sensitivity is usually the cause of the low iron. Also, on a gluten-free diet, many preservative and additives in packet foods are off the menu. Confirmation that their symptoms are due to gluten is discovered when reintroduction of gluten causes a setback.

The benefits are due to a more strict control of the children

Yes, in other studies, more attention to parenting and more positive time spent with children shows benefits in behaviour.

This certainly occurs when parents spend more time preparing food and making sure that their children are eating well. However, yet again the parents find that any reintroduction of gluten, even tiny amounts, can cause a relapse.

A double-blind randomised control trial is essential

Yes, a randomised control study is a very good way to get objective results. This type of study is the mainstay of much medical research, especially for drug trials. Briefly, in such a study the patients would be randomly split into two groups. One group would get gluten-free foods; the other group would get gluten-containing foods. The group into which you are allocated to is kept a secret from both you and the study observers until the end of the trial.

In my opinion, the reports from the affected families are so strong that it is unreasonable to knowingly deprive someone of the very real benefits of a gluten-free diet. However, in the future this experiment needs to be done to convince the sceptics. The irony is that those who are already convinced do not want to cause any more distress to their patients. But on the other hand, the sceptics are unwilling to do experiments in a field in which they lack belief. This stalemate has gone on for years.

The patients would have got better anyway

Yes, perhaps some of these people might get better anyway. But most come to see me following months, or years of illness and suffering. After a full medical assessment and blood tests, if they seem to be gluten-sensitive, I commence them on a three-month gluten-free diet. The astonishing fact is that most of these people get better within weeks (the younger the person, the more quickly they improve). If this response was to happen occasionally, then it might be coincidence. But these "cures" can be seen time and again with a gluten-free diet. Again, if they infringe, then they relapse.

Gluten-free is a big imposition on these families

I disagree. Previously, I also thought that a gluten-free diet was a major burden. I have gone on a gluten-free diet for several months and some of my family are strictly gluten-free. In my experience, a gluten-free diet is not a difficult diet to follow. Yes, it does take extra time, money and commitment. But it is not complex. Few children rebel against it. The adults are relieved to at last be on a program that gives them a new life. Nowadays, there are so many good gluten-free products which are widely available. The first few weeks are the most difficult.

In my experience, people usually eat more healthily on a gluten-free diet. To overcome the initial difficulties, we have written a starter book that explains the diet in a straightforward manner, *Going gluten-free: how to get started*. A gluten-free diet is now relatively easy. Carrying it on for years and years is where it can be more challenging. There are also some social drawbacks – but these are nothing compared with the benefits.

Any diet works

I disagree. Many of my patients have tried many other sorts of diets without the relief that they have been searching for. Once the diagnosis of *The Gluten Syndrome* has been made, then they find it much easier to follow the new food restriction. They feel better at last.

The IgG-gliadin is a non-specific test

I disagree. I have been investigating the IgG-gliadin test for over ten years. Usually, if someone has symptoms, and they have a high IgG-gliadin antibody level, then they will respond favourably to a gluten-free diet. On the other hand, if they have a normal IgG-gliadin, they usually do not respond. However, this is not always the case. Unfortunately, many laboratories are now discontinuing the IgG-gliadin test because it is not diagnostic of coeliac disease. However, the widespread community recognition of gluten-sensitivity will turn this tide. I predict that soon every laboratory will start testing for IgG-gliadin antibodies again.

The brain damage concept is pure speculation

I disagree. I believe that I have argued my case well. There is strong evidence from a wide source of medical information: from patient symptoms; from neurological clinics; from brain scan studies; from post mortems; from nerve cell histology; from brain cell physiology; and from the amazing responses on a gluten-free diet. The brain and nerve tissues are responsible for the regulation of all of your body's functions. When this neurological control goes wrong, you can develop a myriad of symptoms such as are experienced in *The Gluten Syndrome*.

Comments from medical reviewers

I have submitted a number of gluten-sensitivity papers for medical peer review. Here are some of their comments.

"The whole study is an open-label, retrospective, not blinded investigation, based not on objective findings but only on parents and children's subjective report. The magnitude of placebo effect is likely to be huge and to exert an unacceptable influence on the author's conclusions."

"A rather preposterous claim is presented by the author in the discussion. In fact, if it is true that anti-gliadin IgG are markers of gluten sensitivity (to the point of requiring a gluten-free diet!) it can be concluded that 10% of the world population must be gluten-sensitive and should require a diet".

"Overall this study is an interesting observation but until an appropriate prospective randomised control trial is performed with some objective measures of compliance with diet and outcome, the interpretation of this data remains speculative."

"How was clinical improvement measured? Unless there are some objective or at least semi-objective measures the statement of improvement carries little weight."

"All patients were placed on a gluten free diet irrespective of the biopsy results. This was not conducted as part of a clinical trial with a finite time frame: rather it was standard practice. I don't think it is justifiable putting people on gluten-free diets unless they have proven coeliac disease. This practice creates major difficulties sorting out the question of coeliac disease down the track. In addition the practice reported herein is contrary to the current recommendations for the diagnosis and management of coeliac disease."

"The author persists in the use of screening tests (anti-gliadin antibodies) which are now considered defunct by most because of the poor sensitivity and specificity compared to tTG and EMA."

"It comes as no surprise that the biopsy positive and tTG positive groups respond to the diet, as the majority have coeliac disease or coeliac disease 'in waiting'. "

"But the negative group is difficult to interpret. These patients are likely not to have coeliac disease (>95%) but still responded to the diet. The effect may well be placebo but conclusions here are difficult without a control group treated with the diet, e.g. a group with anti-gliadin negative but with GI symptoms."

"The major study outcome was response to diet but the information is derived by history alone in a retrospective chart review. No other measures of response were undertaken such as a standardised questionnaire."

Now it is my turn to respond to these reviewers.

Rebuttal of the medical reviewers

I expect scientific reviews to be objective. Here are some of my rebuttals to the reviewers.

"The reviewer states: *"I don't think it is justifiable putting people on gluten-free diets unless they have proven coeliac disease."* This is the reviewer's opinion. However it is irrelevant to the paper. It attacks my practice and ignores the data. The purpose of this paper is to show that children on a gluten-free diet do improve, despite not having coeliac disease. The reviewer has rejected the concept of the paper, not the data."

"The reviewer states: *"This practice creates major difficulties sorting out the question of coeliac disease down the track."* This statement is not correct and is made with only coeliac disease in mind. The point of the paper is to show that those children who do not have coeliac disease frequently improve on a gluten-free diet. However, later the reviewer agrees that the group of interest are very unlikely to have coeliac disease."

"The reviewer states: *"The practice reported herein is contrary to the current recommendations for the diagnosis and management of coeliac disease".* The reviewer rejects the concept of the paper. The basis of this research was to look outside the guidelines. Progress cannot be made by being constrained by the status quo. In the paper I clearly state that the gluten guideline was contested. How can the guidelines be challenged when staying within the guidelines?"

"The reviewer states: *"The author persists in the use of screening tests (anti-gliadin antibodies) which are now considered defunct by most because of the poor sens/spec compared to tTG."* This shows a lack of understanding about the purpose of the audit. The central point of the paper is to use the anti-gliadin antibodies as a *diagnostic* test for gluten-sensitivity. In the paper I state that the anti-gliadin antibodies are not a good test for coeliac disease. But this paper is not about coeliac disease. It is about children reacting to gluten who do not have coeliac disease."

"The reviewer states: *"It comes as no surprise the positive biopsy group and the positive tTG groups respond to the diet as the majority have coeliac disease or coeliac disease in waiting."* The reviewer accepts the improvement in these two groups without demanding a control group for these two groups."

"But the reviewer then says: *"Interpretation of the positive anti-gliadin and negative tTG group is difficult. These patients are likely not to have coeliac disease but still responded to the diet. The effect may well be placebo but conclusions here are difficult without a control group".* I agree that a control group would be of benefit. However, this audit shows that by parental report, the response to gluten-free diet in this group is similar to those in the coeliac or possible coeliac group. A placebo response of 84% is improbable. This would also infer that the benefits of a gluten-free diet for the coeliacs is also attributable to a placebo response rather than to an improvement in their disease."

"The reviewer states: *"The major study outcome was response to diet but the information is derived by history alone in a retrospective chart review."* Being retrospective does not negate the response of the parents. Clinical history was taken using a structured interview style. A formal standardized questionnaire would be of little additional benefit. The responses to the gluten-free diet were recorded verbatim from the parent."

"The reviewers invoke the placebo effect to dismiss these disturbing results. I am not alone in recognizing children with *The Gluten Syndrome*. There is a vast amount of data in the literature showing that gluten can cause symptoms over and above coeliac disease."

What the patients say

Gluten Syndrome stories

You have read what the critics and reviewers say, and you have read my rebuttals. Now it is the turn of the families to say how *The Gluten Syndrome* has affected them and tell you their experiences with gluten. For each person I give their blood tests and biopsy findings. The IgG-gliadin is high if it reads above 20 units. The HLA result for DQ2/DQ8 is given if they had this test. They are presented to you by age order.

Lauren, 1 year 3 months.
IgG-gliadin 33; IgA-gliadin 4; tTG 3; no biopsy; HLA positive.

Lauren has been gluten-free for two months and now Mum says what she was like before she was gluten-free, how she is now, and how long it took her to get better. Mum said:

> "Lauren had constant diarrhoea. She was quite grumpy and grizzly at night. She had eczema. She was still a happy child but she wasn't as happy as she is now. We are now two months down the track and we noticed a difference within the first three weeks. Her poos got more solid, she didn't grizzle as much during the night with sore tummies. If she has gluten we really know about it now, especially in the afternoons. She is very grizzly all night. She doesn't necessarily wake up but she is grizzling and rolling her self into a little ball.
>
> Her eczema has gone down. Her skin is not nearly as rough. She didn't have severe eczema but she had enough that her skin didn't look as nice as a baby's could. That's gone. Her poos are more solid, they are a better colour, and they are not as white as they used to be. She is a happy, healthy little girl".

Angus, 3 years.
IgG-gliadin 142; IgA-gliadin 10; tTG 12.
Biopsy eosinophilic oesophagitis, normal small bowel.

Angus was having tummy pains and grumpy. His was short.
He had some egg allergy with eczema.

He often refused meals and was lethargic and irritable. He was
sick tired and grumpy! Mum said:

"Angus went gluten-free two weeks ago, after the biopsy. I
think it was 4 to 5 days when we noticed a difference that he
wanted to eat his meals, he was hungry, he was asking for
food. He wasn't lying on the couch.

He could run around with his brother. He is not yet one
hundred percent, but definitely it is such a vast improvement
that my husband and I have noticed.

Before this we were just putting Angus' behaviour down that he
was being naughty around food. Every time a meal came he
would play up and not be at the table and not want to eat. But
it's nice to know it is actually some thing wrong with him and he
was in pain.

My husband didn't use to come home until after meal times
were over because it was such a stressful time to arrive in the
house. But now he comes home and Angus is happily eating
his tea, so it is quite nice".

Ben, 4 years.
IgG-gliadin 67; IgA-gliadin 22; tTG 9.
Biopsy normal; HLA negative.

Mum said:

"Ben was always tired and unwell, Now that he is gluten-free he is bouncing with energy. He is happy again! I took Ben to the doctors so many times. He was always so very tired and got ill lots. I thought it could be an allergy so I asked my doctor to see an allergy specialist – that's how we got to see Doctor Rodney Ford. He listened to what I had to say, I felt valued and heard.

He said we have different options to try, it was very encouraging. First of all Ben had to have some blood tests. They came back showing that he was gluten sensitive.

He went gluten-free and within days he was different. His energy levels increased so much it was like he was hyperactive because he never had so much energy in his life before. I felt bad that I had made him sick all this time by feeding him gluten. But I was relieved that we had at last found out now.

We are now six months down the track. He is used to his energy and is enjoying sports so much more, which my husband is very pleased about. Before changing his diet he would just like to play quiet indoor games.

My husband and I both recently had a cold and Ben, for the first time didn't get it! He is also growing taller all the time and really looking well and happy now. We are so relieved that at last he is happy and healthy again. Who would have thought that gluten could cause all of this!" Sarah (thankful mother).

Ella, 4 years
IgG-gliadin 9; IgA-gliadin 4; tTG 3; no biopsy.

Mum and Dad said:
"Ella was a screamer from the word go. She was diagnosed as having both colic and reflux.

At 7 months she was introduced to solids. Her weight gain slowed down which concerned us. Ella became unsettled and irritable again with the change in diet. Ella continued to be an irritable little girl and tantrums were a regular part of her behaviour.

At 18 months of age she began getting regular fevers. She would eat very little during this time and refused to eat for a couple of days afterwards. During this time she lost a lot more weight and had no energy. Doctors advised us that it was more likely to be a virus. She had some blood tests because of our concerns – these came back clear. A dairy intolerance was suggested. This was our thought, but we wanted confirmation from a medical professional.

Through a family contact we found out about Doctor Rodney Ford. By the time of our first appointment she had been gluten-free for two weeks and we had noticed significant improvement in her behaviour and a return of appetite. Dr Ford spent a lot of time with us listening to our story. He wanted her to stay on a gluten- and dairy-free diet for three months and then we would reassess. He thought that she was most likely gluten-sensitive and ordered another set of blood tests.

We were relieved to finally talk to a medical professional who was admitting that food was most likely the cause of our little girl's problem. At the end of the three month period Ella is a totally different little girl. She is happy, content and appears to have a lot more energy. She at last put on some weight. This proved to us that even though the medical tests showed that her levels were normal her little body wasn't coping with the food she was eating.

We have noticed that when she accidentally has something with gluten in it, she becomes upset and feverish within an hour or so. She also wakes several times during the night screaming. It is a great relief to us to have a diagnosis for Ella and to know that now she is able to live the life of a happy wee girl.

We have found it very frustrating at times trying to reach this point as a lot of the medical professionals we have seen have been very reluctant to confirm our thoughts that food was the problem." Brendon & Alison.

Cole, 5 years.
IgG-gliadin 22; IgA-gliadin 5; tTG 5.
No biopsy.

Cole had severe eczema. Mum tells about what happened before and after Cole went gluten-free. Mum said:
"He was very itchy and rashy all over. He was very uncomfortable, scratching his eczema until it was bleeding. He was cranky and tired as well. We tried various creams and diets and things but they did not seem to help. Then we came to see Dr Rodney Ford, and had a blood test. He has a high gluten test and low iron. Cole went gluten-free and by 3 months his skin was better. Now he is comfortable, smooth skin, and just a little bit of moisturising needed instead of heaps of hydrocortisone cream."

Dad said, "He wasn't concentrating and then within weeks of going gluten-free other people (unprompted people) asked "what have you done with Cole he is concentrating a lot more?" and they noticed the change in him without us saying that we had been to see Dr Ford or anything. So, that was a big thing for us. Now when he has gluten his eczema gets worse and he gets a sore tummy."

Blaire, 6 years.
IgG-gliadin 30; IgA-gliadin 37; tTG 7.
Biopsy normal.

Mum said:
"In hindsight, the trouble began when Blaire was rushed to hospital at the age of 14 weeks with acute abdominal pain. But as she got older, she began to have more and more episodes of stomach pain – to the point that from the age of 5 years she would just drop to the floor, all of a sudden in extreme pain, clutching her stomach and crying. It could happen anywhere in a supermarket, at home, and it was debilitating. There was nothing that we could do.

Now she has been gluten-free for over a year and she enjoys being gluten-free. She doesn't stress about it at all. She doesn't feel as if there is anything she is missing out on.

She has said that she is actually scared of gluten, the same way that I am scared of bee stings because I am allergic to them. Blaire is scared of gluten because of the pain that she would have to endure. And that keeps her on the diet.

Since she has been off all gluten there is no tummy pain whatsoever. She is just a happy, normal child without any incidents at all. Her skin has improved dramatically. She had very dry, skin on her arms and legs. The skin around her fingernails isn't ripping as much, and she is much more settled in her mood."

Melissa, 6 years.
IgG-gliadin 106; IgA-gliadin 15; tTG 4; HLA positive.
Biopsy eosinophilic oesophagitis, normal small bowel.

Melissa has eosinophilic oesophagitis. This was consistent with her symptoms of abdominal pain and reflux. She used to cry every night. Her sore tummies were attributed to behaviour problems. She now recognizes that she reacts to eating gluten. Mother said:

"She had a weetbix in the morning. By that evening she was in severe pain in the stomach. By the next morning, she was on the toilet with diarrhoea. Another time I made muffins for Melissa with a low gluten bread mix and that gave her a sore stomach. Now she is gluten-free she doesn't get any more tummy pains and has more energy."

Caitlin, 7 years.
IgG-gliadin 33; IgA-gliadin 8; tTG 5; no biopsy.

Mum said:

"Before Caitlin went on this gluten-free diet she was extremely car sick, that why she was referred to a paediatrician (Dr Rodney Ford). She got sick within one block, with no windy roads. She would be vomiting and look very white. She got very sick. She was also having headaches at school, pain behind the eyes, vomiting, and she would come home and then vomit a few more times and sleep for about 12 hours. This was happening quite often. About once a week she would have one episode of this, like a migraine, sore headache and vomiting. She was unhappy at school, she was having up and down moods and generally irritable.

Now Caitlin is gluten-free she is not getting car sick, and she has only told me about one headache in the last four months – and she didn't vomit with it. So her migraines have gone, her car-sickness has gone and she is happier at school. She got an award for good work habits, and always applying herself well at school. And her behaviour has just been excellent.

We can see that the gluten-free diet, has made a big difference to Caitlin, and she knows it too. Because she won't go off the gluten-free diet, because she says "mummy, I will get sick again". And she feels really well on the gluten-free diet. So she is almost stricter than I am about it. She knows that she is a lot better."

Petra, 8 years.
IgG-gliadin 159; IgA-gliadin 35; tTG 5; HLA negative.
Biopsy normal, low disaccharidase enzymes.

Petra said:
"I get a sore tummy when I eat gluten things. That's really annoying. Bring on gluten-free for me! When I started I didn't want to eat gluten-free. When mum and I went shopping first, I thought "yuck!" But when I tasted it, it was yum. So we started getting lots of gluten-free foods.

My favourite is mum's chocolate brownie. Now we have lots of things I like. But I still can't eat lots of things I like too. The things I like very much are – chocolate brownies, banana splits, egg rolls, pancakes, corn fritters, some GF bread and biscuits, toasties, GF noodles and popcorn. Father Christmas gave me a smoothie maker and an ice-cream maker. Now I have lots of drinks, smoothies, milk shakes, fluffy milk and ice-cream too.

We also made a nice Christmas cake. We made the same recipe two ways, one with gluten-free flour and one with a hazelnut meal instead of flour. This one tasted great – it was nicer texture than the flour although it was a little crumbly."

Esther, 9 years.
IgG-gliadin 37; IgA-gliadin 55; ttG 11; EMA negative.
No biopsy.

Esther had constipation, abdominal pain, and a poor appetite.
Mum said:
"We found out that Esther was gluten intolerant at Christmas
time. We have taken her off gluten. Esther had a lot of trouble
with her bowels, a lot of trouble passing her motions and we
found that it has taken about 3 or 4 months for her to get better.
Now we don't have any problems, we don't have any messes
on her underwear because that used to happen a lot and she
can now actually pass the motion.

I found that she has a lot more energy which is really good.
Her skin is coming right as well. The skin on her chest and
back was very dry and scaly and that has come right. When
she had some gluten by mistake (in a sausage), Esther said,
"Within about an hour my tummy was so sore, I felt like being
sick, but I didn't spew up. Gluten is not very good for me!"

Ellen, 10 years.
IgG-gliadin 31; IgA-gliadin 4; ttG 8; HLA negative.
No biopsy.

Ellen came to see me because of her sore tummy aches,
headaches, back aches and slow growth. She was often waking
up with pain and frequently had time off school. She has a
brother with autistic spectrum disorder and another brother who
has diabetes and coeliac disease. Ellen said:
"I had sore stomachs, diarrhoea, sore back, headaches, but now
I am on gluten-free I feel much better. I have had sore
stomachs only twice, but that was because I was silly and ate
some gluten! No back pain, very rare headaches, and I feel a
hell of a lot better!"

Tessa, 12 years.
IgG-gliadin 30; IgA-gliadin 5; tTG 5.
No biopsy.

Tessa said:
"Before, I had really sore stomachs and in the morning. I would like get acidy stuff in my throat and I would have either really loose poos or really hard. At school I would feel sick all the time, like I noticed from when I was younger. When I think about it now, I always had sore stomachs. And at night I would be really tired. I would be crashing like at 7.30 pm on the couch and falling asleep.

Then, I went gluten-free about three months ago. I feel so much better. I have so much more energy, like I can stay up heaps longer and didn't have any sore stomachs, no indigestion, or heart burn. It's great. The diet is a bit of a pain, but I am really adjusting to it. It's getting easier."

Ben, 12 years.
IgG-gliadin 22; IgA-gliadin 9; tTG 11.
No biopsy.

Mum said:
"Since Ben has been gluten-free for the last 6 weeks he has been just like a new person, really. We have now noticed that Ben's bad reactions to gluten have happened with jelly (through a neighbour giving him jelly without realizing, and when we read the packet that had wheat in it). So obviously, a minute trace of gluten seems to upset him – you know about it the next day! It basically writes off his whole day!"

He went to stay with his grandmother and she was fantastic. She went out and got everything gluten-free and Ben thought it was wonderful. But he had a really bad day – he just wouldn't want to do anything. He was back to the state how he was beforehand. Grandma declared, "No I haven't given him anything at all with gluten in it", but when she pulled out a Vita-fresh juice packet she said "this was the only thing", and she looked at it and it had wheat in it. We think that is what it caused Ben the problem.

Ben said:
"Oh yeah, I guess I don't feel like running around and doing things when I have gluten. When we were up at our batch I was able to do runs, but sometimes I didn't feel like running after I had that gluten stuff. Also, I didn't feel like eating anything."

Anna, 16 years.
IgG-gliadin 81; IgA-gliadin 13; EMA negative.
Biopsy normal.

Anna's main symptoms were tiredness and abdominal pain. An adult gastroenterologist did not suggest a gluten-free diet. However, by instinct she began to go on a low gluten diet. It wasn't until she went strictly gluten-free did she get the result she was looking for. I asked her what happens when she eats gluten and how quickly she experienced symptoms. Anna replied:

"Sometimes, if I eat a lot of gluten, my symptoms can come on straight away – that is within a few minutes. Otherwise, if I only have only a little bit, I feel sick and these symptoms will come on about an hour or so later. I get a sore stomach, like nausea and stuff, and a headache sometimes. It can take up to an hour or so for this to all go away.

A gluten-free diet is annoying. Especially, when I go out with friends because I can't eat what they are eating. But if I do eat it, then the gluten makes me feel sick. I feel better that I am not eating gluten at the moment."

Rebecca, 17 years.
IgG-gliadin 54; IgA-gliadin 4; tTG 3; EMA negative.
Biopsy normal; HLA negative.

"Hey, my name is Rebecca and I am 17 years old. I have had stomach pain and headaches for a long time. I remember going to the doctor frequently when I was at primary school. But it was at intermediate school, when I was 11, that the stomach pain started to get quite severe. I continued to go to the doctor and when I started to go to High school I had some blood tests done. They showed I was anaemic and my IgG-gliadin antibodies were high.

I was referred to a gastroenterologist and had a gastroscopy which didn't show any evidence of coeliac disease. At times the stomach pain was very severe and I lost a lot of weight (I wasn't very big to begin with). My school kilt had to be taken in 3 inches at the waist and was still too big for me.

The pain affected my ability to play netball which I love and meant I couldn't leave the house without taking a lot of painkillers with me. Sometimes I found it difficult to eat because of the pain and it kept me awake at night. It also affected my schooling as I needed days off and I had trouble concentrating and I didn't have a lot of energy. Over quite a few years the specialist ordered more tests as I was getting worse. I had ultrasound of my abdomen and pelvis, a small bowel barium follow through, a nuclear med scan, a colonoscopy and laparoscopy and numerous blood tests.

The colonoscopy and the laparoscopy were the most uncomfortable and painful. Nothing was conclusive although it did show that there was some sort of inflammatory stuff going on. I went to Dr Rodney Ford and he suggested I try a gluten-free diet. I have been quite strict about my diet and I started to

155

notice that I had less stomach pain after about 2 weeks. By 3 months I had noticed a big improvement. It is now about 7 months since I have been gluten-free and I hardly notice any pain. I am able to play sport and I can go out without taking painkillers with me. My school work has improved and I've needed very little time off school. I can plan to do things without having to worry about coping with pain.

I recently went to a camp where they told me they would provide me with gluten-free food. I started to get some of the old pain back, and when I checked with the cook, the food was low gluten and *not* gluten-free. Since going gluten-free I have had no episodes of severe pain like I used to and I have a normal life. I wish I had done it years ago."

Sonia, 31 years.
IgG-gliadin 28; IgA-gliadin 3; EMA negative.
No biopsy; HLA positive.

Sonia said:
"I have arthritis in the spine. For some reason when I take gluten it seems to affect the arthritis and inflames it and I have to take anti-inflammatories daily and I can't even take a day off. Now I am gluten-free I do not take any medications at all. So, it is perfect!"

Mark, 33 years.
IgG-gliadin 78; IgA-gliadin 10; ttG 12 units; EMA negative.
No biopsy.

I asked Mark to tell me what he is like off gluten and what happens when he does take gluten. He said:
"If I do have foods with a lot of gluten, especially bread and sandwiches at breakfast or for lunch, then I most definitely have headaches by 3.00 pm. I have been used to that. I have

been getting headaches probably most days for the last 3–4 years. I used to take 2–3 paracetamol a day, especially at night.

I am now off gluten. If I don't have gluten then I don't get headaches. Previously, I thought it was always a lack of water, dehydration. But it is most definitely gluten that causes me these headaches. There is no doubt about it."

Michael, 36 years.
IgG-gliadin 80; IgA-gliadin 25; tTG 24; EMA negative.
No biopsy.

Michael had migraines as a child. Michael tells us how he was before he went gluten-free and how he is now. And what happened when he had fish and chips. Michael saaid:
"Prior to going gluten-free I had extensive headaches, probably 3 to 5 days a week. I felt lethargic and had no energy.

Then, 6 months ago I had some blood tests and was advised by Dr Rodney Ford to go gluten-free. I did and it took about 3 months from going gluten-free to becoming fully right. But after that 3 months period the headaches certainly rescinded to almost virtually nil now. I have a lot more energy! Our whole family eats gluten-free

If I do have an accidently have gluten (which doesn't happen very often but it did occur recently, when I had some chips from a take-away shop), the next day I have bad headaches again."

You can read lots more stories from fifty children and families, with many more details in: *The book for the Sick, Tired and Grumpy.*

How common is *The Gluten Syndrome*?

As you can see, there are a lot of children who are getting sick from eating gluten. I have presented you with a lot of data, but the question remains: "How common is gluten-sensitivity?"

An estimate of the incidence of *The Gluten Syndrome* has been calculated using the data in the table below. This calculation is based on the 410 children who responded to a gluten-free diet, the number of responders in each patient category, and the known incidence of coeliac disease (about 1 in 100).

Looking at the table, there were 31 children with coeliac disease compared to 343 '*Not* coeliac' who responded to the gluten-free diet. That is a difference of more than tenfold. In other words, non-coeliac gluten-sensitivity was seen ten times more frequently than coeliac disease.

Calculation of the occurrence of *The Gluten Syndrome*

Patient group	Numbers who responded to a gluten-free diet (n = 410)	Proportion in comparison to definite coeliac	Estimated population incidence
Definite coeliac	31	31:31 = 1	1 in 100 (from research studies)
Possible coeliac	36	31:36 = 1.16	1 in 100
Not coeliac	343	31:343 = 10	**1 in 10**

The logical conclusion is that if gluten-sensitivity occurs at ten times the rate of coeliac disease, and if coeliac disease affects one in every hundred people, then *The Gluten Syndrome* (which includes coeliac disease) must occur in more than one in ten of the population.

Yes! *The Gluten Syndrome* affects at least one in every ten people.

7. The gluten revolution

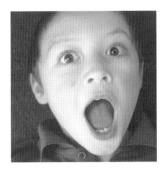

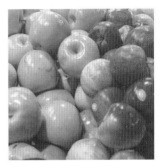

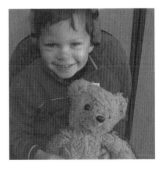

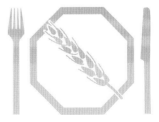

7. The gluten revolution

"Every truth passes through three stages before it is recognized.
In the first, it is ridiculed,
In the second, it is opposed,
In the third, it is regarded as self-evident."
Arthur Schopenhauser

These are turbulent times for gluten. Several years ago, few people knew what gluten was, let alone what it could cause. Now the word 'gluten' can be found in every restaurant, café and supermarket. People are turning to a gluten-free diet in droves. Why is this so?

Are you sick and tired of feeling sick and tired?

The simple answer is that a significant proportion of people who go on a gluten-free diet feel heaps better. They enjoy their new found energy, and are glad to feel well again. My patients talk about a miracle cure. They express relief when, at long last, they feel well again after a decade or more of sickness and frustration.

My hope is that this book might have finally given you the answers that you have been looking for. Eating gluten might be the cause of all your health problems. If you are sick and tired of feeling sick and tired, check out your blood tests, and then try going on a gluten-free diet.

Gluten in the diet has been revealed as a major cause of health problems in millions of people who are being harmed by its toxic and immunological effects. My studies, together with the work of many others, have found that about one in ten people are being made sick by eating gluten. You might be one of them.

More and more gluten has been added to our diets over the last hundred years. Our communities have become habituated to gluten. Consequently, we have become blind to its damaging effects. It is of deep concern that the mechanism through which gluten creates so much damage is its impairment of the brain and nerves.

Why a revolution?

There are huge opposing forces in the gluten industry that will try to maintain the 'status quo'. Consumers are beginning to embrace the gluten-free options, but the gradually increasing pressure they are exerting to change the food chain will inevitably invoke systemised opposition aimed at restoring the stability of the existing system. Sometimes the only way to radically change thought and action is by creating a crisis – by a revolution!

When someone becomes separated or divorced, the changes in their relationship have invariably built up slowly over time. Equal and opposite pressures slowly mount as the partners' differences emerge. Both partners know that something is wrong, but they take no action, and just hope for the best. Until a crisis occurs, the status quo is more comfortable than any change. Then the crisis arrives, and it proves to be a tipping point. A revolution takes place, and a big change occurs – either separation or reconciliation. There is no middle ground.

The medical dilemma

The practice of medicine is driven by conservatism, which engenders a resistance to change. Nowadays, change in the medical field can only be driven by scientific evidence based on ever-more-randomised controlled trials. But how much more evidence is required in support of *The Gluten Syndrome*? What levels of evidence will be required for *The Gluten Syndrome* be considered a respectable diagnosis?

"First do no harm." This is the medical mantra that echoes from the Hippocratic Oath, which contains the statement, "I will carry out regimen for the benefit of the sick and will keep them from harm and wrong." Hippocrates (460-370 BC)

For thousands of years there has been a tension between conservatism (doing what you already know) and experimentation (trying new and untested treatments). Further, these experimental treatments had a tendency to only be tried in extreme circumstances, as a last resort when the patient was near death. I remember when, early in my paediatric career, the newborn premature baby was seen as a huge medical challenge. How could we keep these tiny lives from slipping away? Back then, we did not have much experience in ventilating these small babies, and it was considered almost a death sentence to connect such a baby onto the ventilator, a breathing machine. But we did. Some lived, but many died. Nowadays, aggressive ventilation of these tiny premature babies is routine. Today, it would be unthinkable not to ventilate these babies. It took a lot of trial and error, but in the end, the new idea was triumphant.

Modern medicine has become increasingly complex. Vast amounts of medical information are published on a daily basis. There is a virtual torrent of reports and statistics. How can anyone possibly keep up? The answer is that no one can keep up with everything, and the eventual outcome is that we gradually become more and more specialized in our own fields, while at the same time becoming more and more isolated from each other's knowledge.

Clinical guidelines

A strategy has been devised to try to solve this problem: the development of 'clinical guidelines'. This is a set of suggested rules of treatment and investigation that attempt to distil the most important medical advances, which are then packaged in such a way as to simplify medical decision-making. The theory is that all we have to do is follow these decision-trees, which have been created by committees of experts, and we can feel reassured that we are practicing medicine safely. The downside is, once such a guideline has been established, it becomes a herculean task to alter or replace it. In time it becomes tradition, and then, perhaps, dogma.

Safe medical decisions

The safety of medical decisions is a two-way street. On the one hand, the patient needs to be treated safely so that no harm is done and the patient's condition is managed optimally. On the other hand, the medical practitioner needs the safety of being able to practice without fear of malpractice suits and negligence claims. By strictly adhering to published medical guidelines, the practitioner can sleep peacefully.

When was the last time that you changed a deeply-held belief? How did you feel? Was it during a time of crisis or confusion? Do you see yourself as open-minded? Are you a sceptic? In terms of the gluten arguments, I see no signs that the medical establishment is planning to examine the gluten-sensitivity data with fresh eyes. So it is up to you and your community to make the first moves. This is already happening with the increasing availability of gluten-free foods in shops, cafés and restaurants.

Medical economics

An added complication in all of this is economics. The practice of medicine is becoming increasingly expensive, but there is big money to be made in the medical field, so more and more businesses have been established with a view to profiting from the health industry. Clinical guidelines very much suit this environment. Clinical guidelines can be developed to ensure that the medical workforce acts in a financially prudent way, guided by 'best practice'.

Best practice

What is best practice? Well, it depends on your viewpoint. If you are the patient, you will want everything possible done to ensure your good health, whatever the cost. If you are the doctor, you will want to ensure that your patient gets the best treatment you can provide without any concerns about criticism from either your patient or your colleagues. If you are the manager of a health care organisation, you will want to ensure the most efficient use of resources, which generally means the minimum standard of care that you can get away with.

There are many competing pressures in medicine. Decision making has become a dilemma. Innovation is discouraged, which suffocates progress. The focus of medical guidelines has been to investigate and treat disease, rather than to improve health. New procedures have to be cost-effective. Ignoring people who feel sick, tired and grumpy, but are not ill, can be seen as cost-effective behaviour.

Randomized controlled trial

The holy grail for medical research is the 'double-blind randomized controlled trial'. A randomized controlled trial (RCT) is a scientific procedure used to test the efficacy of medicines or medical procedures. It is considered to be the most reliable form of scientific evidence. This is because it is designed to eliminate the various biases that can so easily compromise the validity of medical research.

Everyone wants to know if a new medicine or a new treatment protocol really works. The person selling the product stands to gain financially and/or professionally by convincing the community that their remedy works, thus the seller is likely to be biased, and prone to exaggerating the effectiveness of the medicine or treatment. In days gone by, biased and overblown claims were often made, and patients often approached the remedy with a degree of scepticism. They were uncertain, but hoped that the medicine or treatment worked. This hope of a cure feeds the placebo effect.

Placebo effect. The placebo effect is the phenomenon whereby people who think that they will get better usually do get better. It can be extremely effective, creating strong bias in favour of a medicine or treatment or, in the context of *The Gluten Syndrome*, towards a particular diet. In psychological terms, it is recognised that we can sometimes become well by 'thinking' ourselves well. So, if we are told that we will improve, and convinced by what we hear, then it is likely that we will indeed get better, whatever the treatment. This effect is regarded by some as a mysterious self-healing force generated by the mind-body connection (it can also work in the opposite way: those who think they will never become well, won't! – this is called the 'nocebo effect').

Surprisingly, the placebo effect has been reported as occurring in up to eighty percent of cases in some circumstances. Therefore, uncontrolled clinical trials and case reports have to be evaluated in this light. As scientific research has progressed, public expectations of unbiased reporting have risen.

The RCT method. The most rigorous method for obtaining evidence for drugs and new procedures is the randomised controlled trial (RCT). This takes the following factors into account:

o   The effects of a particular treatment may be small and t herefore undetectable except when studied systematically over a large population.

o   We humans are incredibly complex. We don't all react to the same stimulus in the same way. This makes inference from single clinical reports unacceptable as scientific evidence.

Some conditions will just spontaneously disappear (this is called remission).

o   The placebo effect, through the simple process of administering the treatment, may have direct psychological effects on us.

It is clear therefore that case reports and open clinical trials, such as the one I reported in Chapter 6, must be viewed with sceptism until such time as sufficient evidence has been gathered. But how much proof is necessary?

Bogged down with information

Over the last decade, medical guidelines have become widely established to treat and manage a wide array of conditions, including coeliac disease. The tendency now is to amass all available data in the form of a 'meta-analysis'. The best-known organisation that does this sort of work is the Cochrane Library. Although this provides a safeguard for both patients and medical practitioners, it also has the effect of stifling new and experimental thinking.

Another problem that stems from these meta-analyses is that they cannot comment on areas that have not yet been carefully studied, for instance gluten-sensitivity. The upshot of all this is that those areas where the data is sparse are conveniently ignored by the medical profession. Such areas are seen as fringe, and are looked upon with suspicion.

No pharmaceutical sponsor

Look around you and you will see that we are surrounded by giant corporations advertising their wares. We are seduced by promises of a better lifestyle, and enticed to buy things that we don't really need, ever-tempted to upgrade to the next level.

The same applies in medicine. The pharmaceutical companies all want to make a profit. The more their drugs are prescribed, the more money they can make. Depression and gastric reflux diseases are common problems, hence they are fertile ground for drugs that purport to offer some benefit. Accordingly, advertising by the manufacturers of these products tends to focus on these conditions, together with the accompanying remedies, and medical practitioners are encouraged to prescribe the remedies offered by these companies.

But where are the big promoters of coeliac disease and gluten reactivity? They're nowhere to be seen! There are no drugs available, and therefore no ongoing benefits to the pharmaceutical industry. Indeed, the opposite is true. *The Gluten Syndrome* is an important – perhaps the major – contributor to cases of depression and gastric reflux. If this was recognized, it is conceivable that millions of people would suffer no more. Their depression and gastric reflux could be eradicated simply by aadherence to a gluten-free diet. Ominously though, it is the pharmaceutical companies who stand to gain the most if knowledge of *The Gluten Syndrome* is denied and suppressed.

Gluten blood tests dumped

Ten years ago, the blood test that was used to help detect coeliac disease was the test that I have referred to as the 'IgG-gliadin' test (more accurately termed the 'anti-gliadin antibody' test). Disappointingly, when results from this test were compared to those from the newer tissue-damage antibody test (the tTG test), the IgG-gliadin test was found to be insufficiently specific to be used to identify coeliac disease patients. Moreover, it was discovered that ten percent of the community had elevated levels of these gliadin antibodies. However, this finding has not been investigated until now.

Because the new tissue-damage blood test proved to be more accurate in detecting the presence of coeliac gut damage, the gluten test was written off as 'non-specific'. Gluten antibody testing is being unceremoniously abandoned by medical laboratories.

However, the gliadin test is being dumped before the pivotal question has been answered: "What is the meaning of a high gliadin antibody level if you do not have coeliac disease?" My research, along with that of many other groups, has shown that the presence of these gliadin antibodies is extremely useful in diagnosing *The Gluten Syndrome*.

Defending the status quo

New ideas always stimulate reactionary thinking. People tend to defend the status quo and resist change. This pattern has been seen throughout the ages, as illustrated by the following milestones in history.

Nicolaus Copernicus (1473-1543) studied medicine and astronomy. His open-minded pondering brought him to the realisation that the earth could not be the centre of the universe. In 1543, he published his completed work *The revolutions of the celestial spheres*. In his proposed system, the Earth was no longer the centre of the universe, but revolved around the sun with the other planets. This was a radical viewpoint, and ran counter to the dogma of the Church. Copernicus's concept was banned by the Catholic Church and remained on the forbidden list until 1835, nearly 300 years later.

Galileo Galilei (1564-1642) was a professor of mathematics who was renowned for perfecting the refracting telescope. This enabled him to detail the movements of the planets. His brilliant research affirmed the truth of the Copernican system with the sun at its centre. In 1632, he presented his findings in *Dialogue on the two principal systems of the world*. This publication was also banned by the Church and Galilei was brought before the Inquisition. Under the threat of torture he recanted, and was placed under house arrest. It was not until 1992, 360 years later, that the sentence passed on him by the Inquisition was formally retracted by the Pope.

Louis Pasteur (1822-1895) put forward the idea that life was not spontaneously created. He showed that the spoiling of food was caused by microbes, and is famous for discovering the technique of short heat treatment used to kill bacteria in milk – the process of 'pasteurization'. Again, his work was initially ridiculed, this time by the scientific establishment.

Joseph Lister (1827-1912) is referred to as the father of antiseptic surgery. He recognised that severe infections were being carried from the autopsy room to the operating room on the hands of surgeons. This cross-contamination was killing patients, including mothers and their newborn babies. Lister's great contribution was the introduction of his antiseptic system in 1867. He soaked his instruments and surgical gauzes in carbolic acid, a well-known disinfectant, but it took another decade before any credence was given to his work and his antiseptic techniques were widely adopted. A speedy acceptance and uptake of this vital knowledge would have saved thousands of lives.

The Helicobacter *pylori* story: Over a hundred years ago, in 1875, German scientists found spiral bacteria in the lining of the human stomach. This bug is now called Helicobacter *pylori*, but at the time of its discovery, it was unable to be grown in culture, and their findings were soon forgotten. Twenty five years later, Professor Jaworski was investigating gastric fluids when he found bacteria with a similarly spiral shape, which he called Vibrio *rugula*.

Jaworski was the first to suggest that this organism might cause gastric diseases, however it was promptly forgotten, and it was not until 1982 that this organism was rediscovered. Two Australian scientists, Robin Warren and Barry Marshall, managed to isolate this organism and, critically, were the first to successfully culture it. In their landmark paper published in 1984, they argued that most stomach ulcers were caused by infection with this bacterium. Previously, gastric upsets and ulcers had been attributed to lifestyle, stress or spicy foods.

Even then, it was not until ten years later, in 1994, that the National Institute of Health published an opinion stating that most recurrent gastric ulcers were caused by H. *pylori*, and it was recommended that antibiotics be included in their treatment. In 2005, Warren and Marshall were awarded the Nobel Prize in Medicine for their work.

Paradigm shift

The journey from the initial discovery of this strange organism, H. *pylori*, to its eventual medical acceptance took over one hundred years! It took that long for the discovery of this bug to be taken seriously and for it to be recognised as the primary cause of peptic ulcers. Ultimately, however, the committee at the Karolinska Institute in Sweden judged this work as the most impacting of its time in medical science. The term for such a revolution in thinking is a paradigm shift.

The time scale of one hundred years is mirrored in the story of gluten, from the first descriptions of coeliac disease to the eventual recognition of *The Gluten Syndrome*. I am not claiming that the recognition of gluten-sensitivity is in the same league as the achievements of the aforementioned scientific giants, however the same resistant forces of tradition and closed-mindedness make it very difficult to persuade people that the accumulation of new information requires the existing pieces of the puzzle to be completely re-evaluated.

The revolution has started

As you can see, the history of science and medicine is littered with vehement arguments against any new idea that runs contrary to traditional beliefs. Ironically however, it takes new ideas to make progress. It was George Bernard Shaw who said that "The reasonable man adapts himself to the world: the unreasonable one persists in trying to adapt the world to himself. Therefore, all progress depends on the unreasonable man."

Even now, medical practitioners are frequently failing to detect patients with coeliac disease, the only entity that they officially recognise as being caused by gluten. Their recognition of coeliac disease is poor. The question is, how much further will they have to be pressed before they come to terms with *The Gluten Syndrome*?

Swell the ranks. Many people are joining the ranks of the gluten revolution. There are thousands of people like you who have read this book and who are concerned about how gluten might be affecting them; there a millions of people who are sick and tired of being ignored and who are looking for more energy and vitality; there are the practitioners in the field of complementary medicine who are aware of the concept of gluten-sensitivity; there are the laboratories who have developed the gliadin antibody test and know that their tests are specific for gluten reactions; there are the gluten-free food manufacturers who have recognised that there is an ever-increasing demand for gluten-free products; there are the networks of people in the health food industry who appreciate the value of high-quality food and a gluten-free diet; and there are the supermarkets and grocery stores that are sensitive to the demands of their customers.

Who might oppose this trend? As previously discussed, medical practitioners are wary of overturning tradition, do not want to be seen as alternative, and want to avoid acting outside of the recommended clinical guidelines. In addition, there are the grain-growers and the bread-makers who make their living from gluten; and the pharmaceutical companies, who make their living from the sick and unwell.

The gluten revolution has well and truly started, and it will prove to be unstoppable. What has been missing up until now is a name that captures the gluten problem. That name is *The Gluten Syndrome*.

The Gluten Syndrome

The big question is, how long will it take for the medical establishment to swallow their pride and agree to seriously and openly examine the facts about gluten reactions (including coeliac disease). There is no key pharmaceutical company championing the cause of gluten, moreover medical scepticism remains high whenever foods are implicated as the possible cause of disease. Scientific truth often flies in the face of tradition, and so I fear that the gluten problem will continue to be ignored, or even suppressed, for a long time yet. In my opinion, the only way forward is by revolution – so let the revolution begin! I have presented my case, and provided you with the evidence.

Blinkered eyes

Unfortunately, the results of the IgG-gliadin blood test have been examined with blinkered eyes, and its relevance has been overlooked. This narrow focus has led to a search for a diagnostic test for coeliac disease without stopping to think about what the gluten blood tests really mean in the wider clinical context.

The approach habitually used by medical professionals to explain away the significance of a positive IgG-gliadin test is to call it 'non-specific', however this is illogical, because this test in fact measures a very specific immunological reaction to gluten.

Conclusion

The Gluten Syndrome refers to the cluster of symptoms that you experience if you react to gluten. It applies to any reaction that is caused by gluten, including coeliac disease and the myriad symptoms that can be experienced throughout your gastro-intestinal tract. It also includes many other symptoms that do not stem from your gut. These include brain and behaviour disorders, irritability and tiredness, skin problems, muscular aches and pains and joint problems.

The Gluten Syndrome affects about one in ten people, however most people who are affected are unaware that their life is being damaged by gluten. Most of the gluten symptoms are most likely to be caused by damage to the nerves and brain. The earlier the problem is identified, the better the response to a gluten-free diet will be.

It turns out that the IgG-gliadin test is a valuable and specific test to identify *The Gluten Syndrome*. Unfortunately however, this test is becoming less widely available.

A strong gluten-free movement is developing globally in response to the knowledge that going gluten-free can be so beneficial to so many people. What has been missing up until now is a name that captures the gluten problem.

The missing name is

The Gluten Syndrome.

8. References

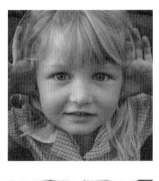

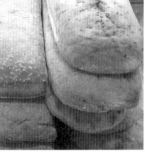

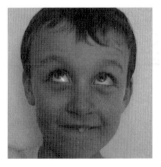

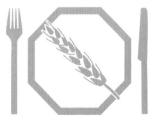

8. References

This is a list of references from research that has been used to support the concept of *The Gluten Syndrome.*

Barker CC, Mitton C, Jevon G, Mock T.
Can tissue transglutaminase antibody titers replace small-bowel biopsy to diagnose celiac disease in select pediatric populations?
Pediatrics. 2005; 115: 1341-6.

Bodé S, Gudmand-Hoyer E.
Symptoms and haematological features in consecutive adult coeliac patients.
Scand J Gastroenterol. 1996; 3: 54-60.

Bonamico M, Mariani P, Thanasi E, et al.
Patchy villous atrophy of the duodenum in childhood celiac disease.
J Pediatr Gastroenterol Nutr. 2004; 38: 204-7.

Bozzola M, Giovenale D, Bozzola et al.
Growth hormone deficiency and coeliac disease: an unusual association?
Clin Endocrinol (Oxf). 2005; 62: 372-5.

Braly, James and Hoggan, Ron.
Dangerous Grains: Why Gluten Cereal Grains May Be Hazardous to Your Health.
Book, 2002. Pub: Penguin Putnam Inc. NY. USA.

Collin P, Reunala T, Pukkala E, et al.
Coeliac disease – associated disorders and survival.
Gut. 1994; 35: 1215-1218.

Collin P, Maki M.
Associated disorders in coeliac disease: clinical aspects.
Scand J Gastroenterol. 1994; 29: 769-775.

Cooke WT, Thomas-Smith W.
Neurological disorders associated with adult coeliac disease.
Brain. 1966; 89: 683-722.

Corazza GR, Andreani ML, Venuro N, et al.
Celiac disease and alopecia areata: report of a new association.
Gastroenterology. 1995; 109: 1333-1337.

Corvaglia L, Catamo R, Pepe G, Lazzari R, Corvaglia E.
Depression in adult untreated celiac subjects: diagnosis by the
pediatrician.
Am J Gastroenterol. 1999; 94: 839-43.

Cronin CC, Jackson LM, Feighery C, et al.
Coeliac disease and epilepsy.
QJM. 1998; 91: 303-308.

Cuomo A, Romano M, Rocco A, et al.
Reflux oesophagitis in adult coeliac disease: beneficial effects of a
gluten free diet. Gut. 2003; 52: 514-517.

De Sanctis A, Addolorato G, Romito A, et al.
Schizophrenic symptoms and SPECT abnormalities in a coeliac
patient: regression after a gluten-free diet.
J Intern Med. 1997; 242: 421-423.

Dicke WK, Weijers HA, Van De Kamer JH.
Coeliac disease II: the presence in wheat of a factor having a
deleterious effect in cases of coeliac disease.
Acta Paediatrica. 1953; 42: 34-42.

Dicke WK.
Coeliac Disease: Investigation of the harmful effects of certain types of cereal on patients suffering from coeliac disease.
MD Thesis. 1950.

Dohan FC.
More on Celiac Disease as a model for schizophrenia.
Biol. Psychiatry. 1983; 18: 561-4.

Duggan J M.
Coeliac disease: the great imitator.
MJA. 2004; 180: 524-526.

Fasano A, Not T, Wang W, Uzzau S, Berti I, Tommasini A, Goldblum SE. Zonulin, a newly discovered modulator of intestinal permeability, and its expression in coeliac disease.
Lancet. 2000; 355: 1518-9.

Fasano A. Regulation of intercellular tight junctions by zonula occludens toxin and its eukaryotic analogue zonulin (review).
Ann N Y Acad Sci. 2000; 915: 214-22.

Fasano A.
Celiac disease – how to handle a clinical chameleon.
N Engl J Med. 2003; 348: 2568-2570.

Fasano A, Berti I, Gerarduzzi T.
Prevalence of celiac disease in at-risk and not-at-risk groups in the United States. Arch Intern Med. 2003; 163: 286-292.

Federico G, Favilli T, Cinquanta L, Ughi C, Saggese G.
Effect of celiac disease and gluten-free diet on growth hormone-binding protein, insulin-like growth factor-I, and insulin-like growth factor-binding proteins.
Horm Res. 1997; 48: 108-14.

Fine KD.
Small Bowel Enteropathy in Patients with Microscopic Colitis: Is It Gluten-Sensitive?
J Clin Gastroenterol. 2001; 32: 193-195.

Fois A, Vascotto M, Di Bartolo RM, Di Marco V.
Celiac disease and epilepsy in pediatric patients.
Childs Nerv Syst. 1994; 10: 450-4.

Fonager K, Sorensen HT, Norgard B, Thulstrup AM.
Cardiomyopathy in Danish patients with coeliac disease.
Lancet. 1999; 354: 1561.

Ford RPK.
Food hypersensitivity in children: diagnostic approaches to milk and egg hypersensitivity.
MD Thesis. 1982. University of New South Wales.

Ford RPK. Who warrants a gluten-free diet?
Royal Australasian College of Physicians (RACP) meeting in Australia, May 2006.
Journal of Paediatrics and Child Health, 2006; 42, A1–A17.

Ford RPK.
Gluten reactions: ten times the celiac problem.
Poster presentation, NASPGHAN, Orlando, Florida, Oct 2006.

Ford RPK.
Sick Tired and grumpy? Who warrants a gluten-free diet?
Poster presentation, NASPGHAN, Orlando, Florida, Oct 2006.

Gale L, Wimalaratna H, Brotodiharjo A, Duggan JM.
Down syndrome is strongly associated with coeliac disease.
Gut. 1997; 40: 492-496.

Gasparrini A, Torre ES, Trivellini C, et al.
Recurrent spontaneous abortion and intrauterine fetal growth
retardation as symptoms of coeliac disease.
Lancet. 2000; 356: 399-400.

Gee S.
On the coeliac affection.
St Bartholomew's Hospital Reports. 1888; 24: 17-20.

Gershon, Michael D.
The Second Brain: a groundbreaking new understanding of
nervous disorders of the stomach and intestine.
Book, 1998. Pub HarperCollins, NY, USA.

Gobbi G.. Coeliac disease, epilepsy and cerebral calcifications.
Brain Dev. 2005; 27: 189-200.

Green PHR, Jabri B.
Coeliac disease.
Lancet. 2003; 362: 383-391.

Hadjivassiliou M, Gibson A, Davies-Jones GAB, Lobo A,
Stephenson T J, Milford-Ward A. Is cryptic gluten sensitivity an
important cause of neurological illness?
Lancet. 1996; 347: 369-371.

Hadjivassiliou M, Gibson A, Grünewald RA, Davies-Jones GAB,
Chattopadhyay AK, Kandler RH, et al. Idiopathic ataxia of late
onset: gluten sensitivity is part of the answer.
J Neurol Neurosurg Psychiatry. 1997; 63: 267.

Hadjivassiliou M, Chattopadhyay AK, Davies-Jones GAB, Gibson
A, Grünewald RA, Lobo AJ. Neuromuscular disorder as a
presenting feature of coeliac disease.
J Neurol Neurosurg Psychiatry. 1997; 63: 770-775.

Hadjivassiliou M, Boscolo S, Davies-Jones GA, Grunewald RA, Not T, Sanders DS, Simpson JE, Tongiorgi E, Williamson CA, Woodroofe NM. The humoral response in the pathogenesis of gluten ataxia. Neurology. 2002; 58: 1221-6.

Hadjivassiliou M, Grunewald RI, Sharrack B, et al. Gluten ataxia in perspective: epidemiology, genetic susceptibility and clinical characteristics. Brain. 2003; 126: 685-691.

Hadjivassiliou M, Grunewald RA, Kandler RH, Chattopadhyay AK, Jarratt JA, Sanders DS, Sharrack B, Wharton SB, Davies-Jones GA. Neuropathy associated with gluten sensitivity. J Neurol Neurosurg Psychiatry. 2006; 77: 1262-6.

Hoffenberg EJ, Emery LM, Barriga KJ, Bao F, Taylor J, Eisenbarth GS, Haas JE, Sokol RJ, Taki I, Norris JM, Rewers M. Clinical features of children with screening-identified evidence of celiac disease. Pediatrics. 2004; 113: 1254-9.

Hoffman, Ronald. Tired All the Time: How to Regain Your Lost Energy. Book, 1993: Pub Poseidon Press.

Holmes GK, Prior P, Lane MR, et al. Malignancy in coeliac disease – effect of a gluten free diet. Gut. 1989; 30: 333-338.

Holmes GKT. Non-malignant complications of coeliac disease. Acta Paediatr. Suppl. 1996; 412: 68-75.

Ghezzi A, Filippi M, Falini A, Zaffaroni M.
Cerebral involvement in celiac disease: a serial MRI study in a patient with brainstem and cerebellar symptoms.
Neurology. 1997; 49: 1447-50.

Illingworth, Ronald S. The normal child: some problems of early years and their treatment.
Book, 1991. Pub. Churchill Livingston. UK.

Lee SK, Green PH.
Endoscopy in celiac disease.
Curr Opin Gastroenterol. 2005; 21: 589-94.

Korn, Danna.
Wheat free, worry-free. The art of happy, healthy gluten-free living.
Book, 2002. Pub: Hay House Inc. CA. USA.

Knivsberg A-M, Reichelt K, Holin T, Nodland M.
A randomised controlled trial of dietary intervention in autistic syndromes.
Nutritional Neuroscience. 2002; 5: 251-261.

Lindh E, Ljunghall S, Larsson K, Lavo B.
Screening for antibodies against gliadin in patients with osteoporosis.
J Intern Med. 1992; 231: 403-406.

Lo W, Sano K, Lebwohl B, et al.
Changing presentation of adult celiac disease.
Dig Dis Sci. 2003; 48: 395-398.

Lowell, Jax Peters.
Against the grain.
Book, 1995. Pub: Henry Holt Co. USA.

Lubrano E, Ciacci C, Ames PR, et al.
The arthritis of coeliac disease: prevalence and pattern in 200 patients.
Br J Rheumatol. 1996; 35: 1314-1318.

Magliocca FM, Bonamico M, Petrozza V, Correr S, Montuori M, Triglione P, Carpino F. Scanning electron microscopy of the small intestine during gluten-challenge in celiac disease.
Arch Histol Cytol.1992; 55 Suppl: 125-30.

Maki M, Collin P.
Coeliac disease.
Lancet. 1997; 349: 1755-1759.

Marks J, Shuster S, Watson AJ.
Small bowel changes in dermatitis herpetiformis.
Lancet. 1966; ii: 1280-1282.

Marsh MN.
The natural history of gluten sensitivity: defining, refining and re-defining.
Q J Med. 1995; 85: 9-13.

Marsh MN. Gluten, major histocompatibility complex, and the small intestine. A molecular and immunobiologic approach to the spectrum of gluten sensitivity ('celiac sprue').
Gastroenterology. 1992; 102: 330-54.

Marti T, Molberg O, Li Q, Gray GM, Khosla C, Sollid LM.
Prolyl Endopeptidase Mediated Destruction of T Cell Epitopes in whole Gluten - Chemical and Immunological Characterization.
J Pharmacol Exp Ther. 2005; 312: 19-26. Epub 2004.

Mercola, Joseph.
The no-grain diet.
Book, 2005. Pub Hodder and Stoughton. USA.

Mills PR, Brown IL, Ojetti V, Sanchez JA, Guerriero C, et al.
High prevalence of celiac disease in psoriasis.
Gastroenterology. 2003; Suppl 1: A656.

Molberg O, Mcadam SN, Körner R, et al.
Tissue transglutaminase selectively modifies gliadin peptides that
are recognized by gut-derived T cells in celiac disease.
Nat Med. 1998; 4: 713-7.

Oberhuber G., Granditsch G., and Vogelsang H.
The histopathology of coeliac disease: time for a standardized
report scheme for pathologists.
Eur J Gastroenterol Hepatol. 1999. 11: 1185-1194.

Parnell NDJ, Ciclitra PJ.
Review article: coeliac disease and its management.
Aliment Pharmacol Ther. 1999; 13: 1-13.

Ranua J, Luoma K, Auvinen A, Maki M, Haapala AM, Peltola J,
Raitanen J, Isojarvi J. Celiac disease-related antibodies in an
epilepsy cohort and matched reference population.
Epilepsy Behav. 2005; 6: 388-92.

Pellecchia M, Scala R, Filla A, De Michele G, et al.
Idiopathic cerebellar ataxia associated with celiac disease: lack of
distinctive neurological features.
J Neurol Neurosurg Psychiatry. 1999; 66: 32-35.

Sbarbati A, Valletta E, Bertini M, et al.
Gluten sensitivity and 'normal' histology: is the intestinal mucosa
really normal? Dig Liver Dis. 2003; 35: 768-73.

Sanders DS, Carter MJ, Hurlstone DP, et al.
Association of adult coeliac disease with irritable bowel syndrome:
a case-control study in patients fulfilling ROME II criteria referred
to secondary care. Lancet. 2001; 358: 1504-1508.

Sjoberg K, Eriksson KF, Bredberg A, et al.
Screening for coeliac disease in adult insulin-dependent diabetes
mellitus. J Intern Med. 1998; 243: 133-140.

Sher K, Mayberry J.
Female fertility, obstetric and gynaecological history in coeliac
disease: a case control study.
Gastroenterology. 1994; 55: 243-246.

Sher KS, Jayanthi V, Probert CSJ, et al.
Infertility, obstetric and gynaecological problems in coeliac disease.
Dig Dis. 1994; 12: 186-190.

Smith, Melissa Diane. Going Against The Grain: How reducing
and avoiding grains can revitalize your health.
Book, 2002. Pub. Contemporary Books. McGraw-Hill N.Y.

Trevisiol C, Ventura A, Baldas V, Tommasini A, Santon D, et al.
A reliable screening procedure for coeliac disease in clinical
practice.
Scand J Gastroenterol. 2002; 37: 679-84.

Troncone R, Greco L, Mayer M, Paparo F, Caputo N, Micillo M.
Latent and potential coeliac disease.
Acta Paediatr. 1996; 412 (suppl): 10-14.

Tursi A.
Gastrointestinal motility disturbances in celiac disease.
J Clin Gastroenterol. 2004; 38: 642-5.

Usai P.
Adult coeliac disease is frequently associated with sacroiliitis.
Dig Dis Sci. 1995; 40: 1906-1908.

Usai P, Usai Satta P, Lai M, Corda MG, Piras E, Calcara C, Boy
MF, Morelli A, Balestrieri A, Bassotti G.
Autonomic dysfunction and upper digestive functional disorders in
untreated adult coeliac disease.
Eur J Clin Invest. 1997; 27: 1009-1015.

Visakorpi JK, Kuitunen P, Savilahti E.
Frequency and nature of relapses in children suffering from the
malabsorption syndrome with gluten intolerance.
Acta Paediatr Scand. 1970; 59: 481-6.

Volta U, De Giorgio R, Granito A, Stanghellini V, Barbara G, et al.
Anti-ganglioside antibodies in coeliac disease with neurological
disorders.
Dig Liver Dis. 2006; 38: 183-7. Epub 2006.

Vogelsang H, Oberhuber G, Wyatt J.
Lymphocytic gastritis and gastric permeability in patients with
celiac disease.
Gastroenterology. 1996; 111: 73-77.

Wills AJ.
The neurology and neuropathology of coeliac disease.
Neuropathol Appl Neurobiol. 2000; 26: 493-6.

Zelnik N, Pacht A, Obeid R, Lerner A.
Range of neurologic disorders in patients with celiac disease.
Pediatrics. 2004; 113: 1672-6.

Natalie's brown bread

This is our favourite bread – it works every time

Place into a bowl the following:
2 cups of warm water *or* milk
1 Tablespoon brown sugar
1 ¼ teaspoon yeast (GF)
1 egg
3 Tablespoons of oil
Approx 500gms GF bread mix (e.g. Healtheries)
  or half bread mix and half baking mix
1 heaped Tablespoon coarse *maize* cornmeal
1 heaped Tablespoon fine *maize* cornmeal *or* rice flour
1 heaped Tablespoon ground linseed
1 heaped Tablespoon sunflower seeds
1 heaped Tablespoon pumpkin seeds [optional]
1 teaspoon guar gum.

Mix ingredients gently together.
Scrape the firmish mixture into your bread maker 'bucket' and cook on the rapid programme with dark crust (some other bread-makers might use the 'basic' programme for best results).

If your bread sinks in centre it may be too moist at the start. You can also use the light crust and large loaf setting for Panasonic bread makers.

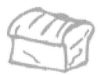

Variations on Natalie's brown bread recipe

This has been our most popular bread – people tell us that it was the breakthrough that they were looking for.

A mum who has just started her gluten-free diet sent us this message:

"I have made this recipe everyday for the last month, and it never fails. My four kids love the bread, and have it as sandwiches in their lunchboxes every day. Their favourite is ham and cheese.

This loaf is slightly sweet but you can adjust the amount of sugar according to taste.

If you make a wetter mixture, then the loaf turns out lighter If the mixture is drier, then the loaf is dense.

I sometimes substitute the Tablespoon of ground linseed and the Tablespoon of sunflower seeds for 2 Tablespoons of LSA meal (ground Linseed, ground Sunflower seeds and blanched Almonds) which is readily available in supermarkets.

This is such a successful bread.

The kids forget that they are eating gluten-free!"

Enjoy!

Other books by Dr Rodney Ford

❑ Eczema! Cure It!

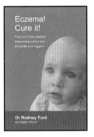

Parents want a cure for their child's eczema! For most, I can help them get their skin back to almost perfect. Find out the secrets! All the information offered in this book is from well-researched approaches to allergy and eczema. Learn how these strategies can help cure your child's eczema. Yes! Eczema can be cured! Find out how!

ISBN 978-0-473-10773-4 (96 pages)
(NZ$24.95 Aus$24.95 US$15.95)

❑ The Gluten Syndrome

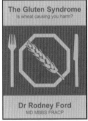

The Gluten Syndrome is the name for the cluster of symptoms that you get when you react to gluten – it can affect your gut, skin and nerves. One in ten people – tens of millions worldwide – are affected but few are aware of this illness. Could this be you?

ISBN 978-0-473-12472-4 (192 pages)
(NZ$34.95 Aus$34.95 US$19.95)

❑ Going Gluten-Free: How to Get Started

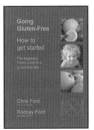

"Overwhelm" is often the first emotion felt when you are confronted by the prospect of a gluten-free diet. Find out how you can get started. Step 1– Get ready: Identify if you really are gluten-sensitive. Step 2 – Get set up: Find out all about gluten. Use our shopping list to help you work out what you can eat. Step 3 – Go gluten-free: Follow the recipes and eating ideas.

ISBN 978-0-473-10491-7 (64 pages)
(NZ$14.95 Aus$14.95 US$9.95)

Available from the website: www.doctorgluten.com

❑ Are You Gluten-Sensitive? Your Questions Answered

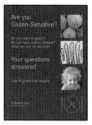

This book is based on the questions that I am so frequently asked by my patients. I answer their questions in detail and put them into the clinical context. There is lots of confusion about the diagnosis and management of people who are gluten-sensitive. This book has been written to clarify this muddle. It is full of practical information.

ISBN 978-0-473-11229-5 (192 pages)
(NZ$34.95 Aus$34.95 US$19.95)

❑ The Gluten-Free Lunch Book

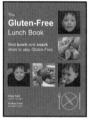

What can I have for lunch? That is our most often asked question. Easy and yummy lunches make all the difference if you are trying to stay gluten-free. We have brought together the best lunch ideas so that you never have to worry about lunch again. Simple and delicious gluten-free lunch box ideas for you and your family. Follow these recipes and eating ideas for a great gluten-free experience.

ISBN 978-0-473-10498-6 (64 pages)
(NZ$14.95 Aus$14.95 US$9.95)

❑ The book for the Sick, Tired & Grumpy

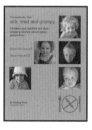

Over 50 people tell their amazing stories. A cure for so many people who feel sick, tired or grumpy. These personal accounts are very moving with a raw honesty that hits home. If you want to feel well and full of energy again – then this book is for you. These children and parents tell about their low energy, their irritability and troublesome symptoms before they discovered their gluten-sensitivity. You then hear how going gluten-free has changed their lives. This might be just the answer you are looking for.

ISBN 978-0-473-11228-8 (192 pages)
(NZ$34.95 Aus$34.95 US$19.95)
Available from the website: www.doctorgluten.com

❑ Full of it! The Shocking Truth About Gluten

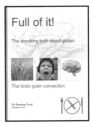

An alarming fact is that gluten can damage your brain. Have you ever wondered why you crave for another hunk of bread? If a food that you ate was slowly eroding the function and the ability of your brain, then would you want to know what that food was? It is gluten! Gluten is linked to ataxia, migraine, ADHD, autism, depression, epilepsy, mood and psychiatric disorders. Gluten also can disrupt your brain's regulation of your gut – causing mayhem in your bowel. Gluten-sensitivity is a brain disease! Read the evidence for yourself.

ISBN 978-0-473-10407-8 (192 pages)
(NZ$34.95 Aus$34.95 US$19.95)

❑ Gluten-Free Parties & Picnics

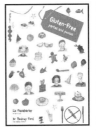

Oh dear, it's Libby's birthday – how will we manage to do a gluten-free party? How will we cope on a family picnic? These questions are answered for your children in a story-book format, in vibrant full colour. It is packed with great party and picnic ideas. Great for your family and friends to learn about the gluten-free issues. It makes it easy for your children to understand about gluten. At last an enchanting gluten book for your children.

ISBN 978-0-473-10774-1 (64 pages, full colour)
(NZ$19.95 Aus$19.95 US$14.95)

Available from the website: www.doctorgluten.com

☐**Eczema! Cure It!**

☐*The Gluten Syndrome*

☐**Going Gluten-Free: How to Get Started**

☐**Are You Gluten-Sensitive? Your Questions Answered**

☐**The Gluten-Free Lunch Book**

☐The book for the **Sick, Tired & Grumpy**

☐**Full of it! The shocking truth about gluten**

☐**Gluten-Free Parties & Picnics**

(Please indicate the number of each book that you want to order. Prices stated on previous page)

Please add postage & handling: 1 book $7.00, 2 books $12, 3 or 4 books $15

(Prices for postage and handling to be paid in the currency of purchase)

Order for:

Name: _____

Postal address: _____

_____

Phone: _____   Fax: _____

Email: _____ @ _____

Number of books required: _____   Currency _____

Cost of books $ _____   Postage $ _____   Total $_____

Method of payment:

Cheque ☐   Visa ☐   MasterCard ☐   (please tick)

Cardholder's name: _____

Credit card number : _____

Signature: _____   Expiry date: _____/_____

Please make your cheque payable to:

Doctor Gluten, PO Box 25-360, Christchurch, New Zealand.

Fax orders: +64 3 377 3605

Email orders: orders@doctorgluten.com

Web orders: www.doctorgluten.com

(Please allow up to 21 days for postal delivery)